THE BIG 15 PALEO COOKBOOK

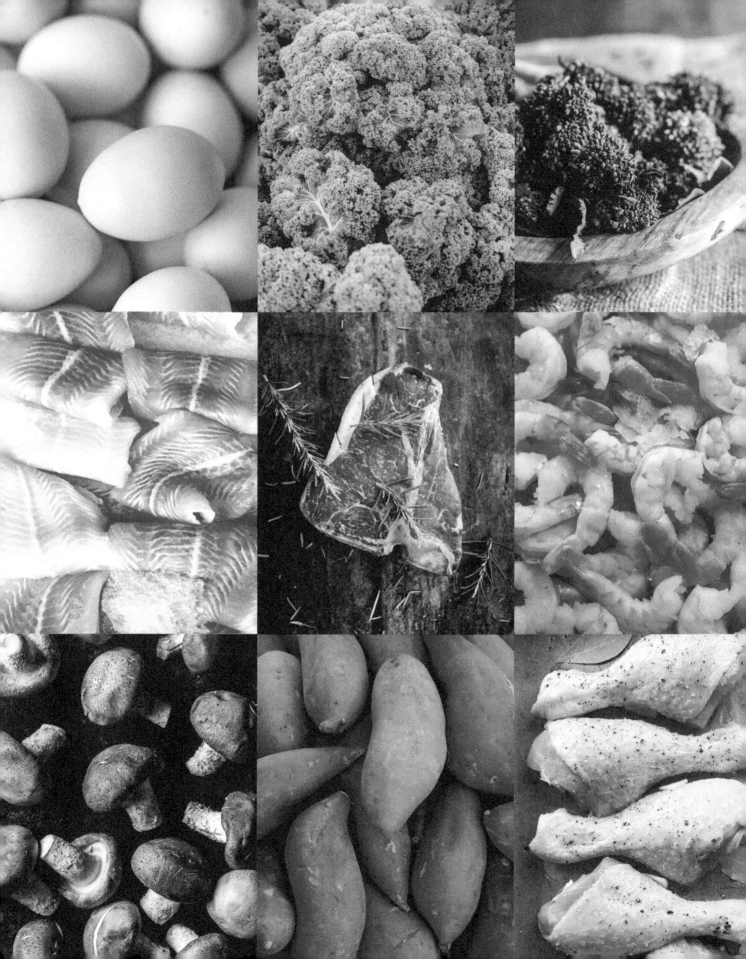

THE
BIG 15
PALEO
COOKBOOK

15 Fundamental Ingredients
150 Paleo Diet Recipes
450 Variations

MEGAN FLYNN PETERSON

R

**ROCKRIDGE
PRESS**

Front cover photography © Stocksy/J.R. PHOTOGRAPHY; Stocksy/Christian B; iStock/flyfloor; Stocksy/Alberto Bogo; Stocksy/Darren Muir; Stockfood/Clive Streeter; Stocksy/Sara Remington

Interior photography © Stocksy/Christian B, p.2, 118; Stocksy/Aniko Lueff Takacs, p.2, 132, Stocksy/Alberto Bogo, p.2, 18; iStock/flyfloor, p.2, 34; Stocksy/J.R. PHOTOGRAPHY, p.2, 48; Stocksy/Sonja Lekovic, p.2, 76; iStock/P_Wei, p.2, 90; iStock/alantobey, p.3; Stocksy/Sara Remington, p.3, 162; iStock/Paulina Lenting-Smulder, p.3, 190; Stocksy/Jeff Wasserman, p.3, 62; Stocksy/Sara Remington, p.6; Stocksy/Darren Muir, p.6; Stocksy/Laura Spinelli, p.6; iStock/Kelly Cline, p.10, 104; Stocksy/Lee Avison, p.10; Stocksy/Gabriel (Gabi) Bucataru, p.10; Stocksy/Carolyn Brandt, p.10; Stocksy/Darren Muir, p.12; Stocksy/Noemi Hauser, p.17; Stockfood/Antti Jokinen, p.23; Stockfood/Ian Garlick, p.41; Stockfood/PhotoCuisine/Thys/Supperdelux, p.57; Stockfood/Gräfe & Unzer Verlag/Klaus-Maria Einwanger, p.71; Stockfood/Tanya Zouev, p.82; Stockfood/Rua Castilho, p.99; Stockfood/Tanya Zouev, p.111; Stockfood/Gräfe & Unzer Verlag/Kramp + Gölling, p.121; Stockfood/Great Stock!, p.139; Stockfood/ Gräfe & Unzer Verlag/Grossmann.Schuerle, p.149; Stockfood/Rua Castilho, p.158; Stockfood/Al MacDonald Partners, LLC, p.167; Stocksy/Tatjana Ristanic, p.183; Stockfood/Clive Streeter, p.197; Stockfood/Mikkel Adsbol, p.205; Stockfood/Charlotte Tolhurst, p.222; Stocksy/Ina Peters, p.230,

Back cover photography © iStock/alantobey; Stocksy/Jeff Wasserman; iStock/P_Wei; Stocksy/Aniko Lueff Takacs

ISBN 978-1-62315-769-2
eBook 978-1-62315-770-8

TO ROB,
WHO BELIEVES IN ME EVEN WHEN I DON'T

Contents

Introduction

I found Paleo at a time in my life when I was otherwise lost.

It was the summer of 2011, I had just moved to a new city, and my life was rife with transition. I was gaining weight, feeling sick, and having trouble getting out of bed in the morning—anxiety and sadness had crept into my day-to-day life, and I wasn't sure how to shake them off. I was eating an almost-vegetarian diet full of dairy and whole grains because I thought that was healthy and balanced, but I wasn't losing weight, my skin was breaking out, my hair was falling out, and I felt sick and dizzy every day.

Sometime around October, my mom mentioned a way of eating that someone at her gym had introduced her to: Paleo—no grains, no dairy, no sugar, no legumes; lots of meat and vegetables, and some fruit. It sounded extreme, especially for someone whose diet consisted mostly of caramel lattes, grilled cheese sandwiches, and vegetarian pasta dishes, but I dove in headfirst and was amazed by the almost-immediate results.

I felt better overall after just seven days. My skin cleared up after a few weeks. I felt calmer and had more energy. After just a month, I had returned to my normal weight and the bald spots on my scalp were filling in with healthy new hair. I began exercising again. And somehow, after what had become a pretty complicated relationship, I was able to start loving food again.

I come from an Italian background, so eating, cooking, and feeding people is in my blood. Some of my favorite memories include my mother in the kitchen, stirring something on the stove, pouring glasses of wine for friends, and setting out huge platters of meat and cheese. My friends always knew not to eat before coming over. When I first went Paleo, I really worried about what a life without pasta might look like, but as I began cutting out processed foods like sugar, grains, and dairy, I learned the power of real food—and that it can be not only vital to our well-being but also delicious and, if I may be so bold, life changing. I may not be rolling out pizza dough these days, but my kitchen is still a place full of love where people gather for great food, friendship, and laughter.

I had always thought of myself as a health-conscious person, but when it came to food, I didn't know where to begin. For a long time, I ate whatever I wanted, felt terrible, and then ran miles to leave behind whatever guilt I was feeling. But when you start with food that gives back to your body, there are no emotional consequences. There is something so empowering about taking charge of your health through nutrition. And it's even better when you can make it happen with delicious and satisfying real food. I feel honored to be sharing these recipes with you.

I hope you find something amazing here.

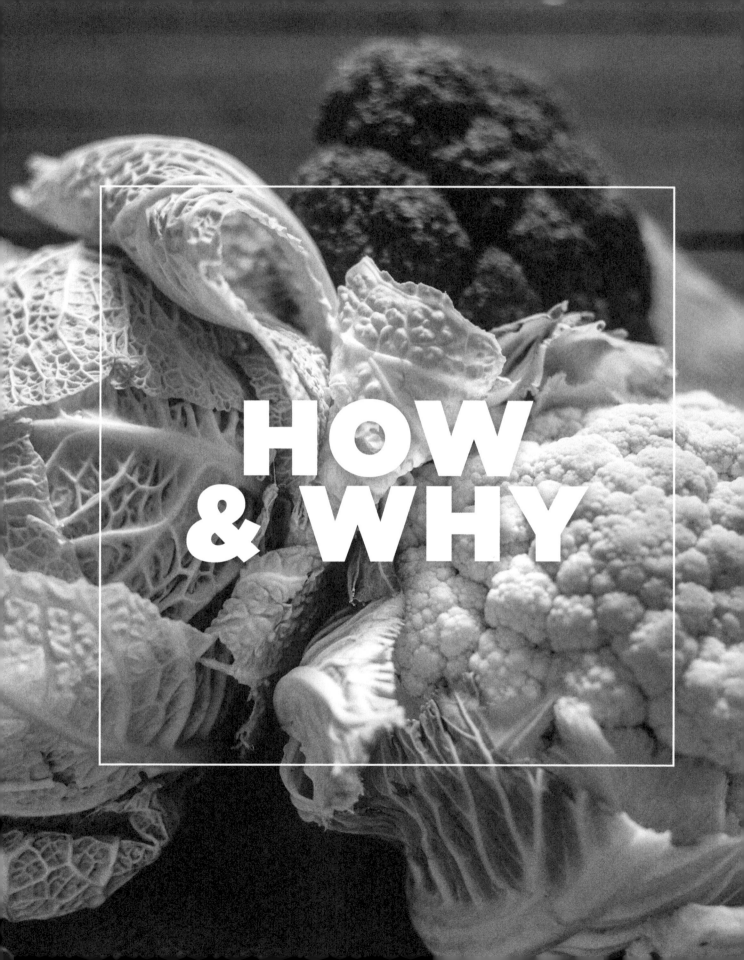

HOW & WHY

The more research you do about Paleo, the more you'll read about organic and grass-fed foods. We've all heard "You are what you eat," and this applies here: By choosing beef that's been raised on grass as opposed to corn, you are maintaining a grain-free diet by extension.

Paleo can be a little tough on a budget, but meal planning will save you so much money in the long run. And I always want to encourage people to just do their best—if you can't afford grass-fed beef or organic vegetables, purchase the best quality that your budget will allow and feel good that you're still making healthy choices.

PALEO, PERSONALLY

My experience with Paleo is just that—my own. People change their diets for any number of reasons, and I always want people to know that you don't have to be feeling terrible, or struggling like I was, to benefit from Paleo. Some people make a switch to Paleo for health reasons, while others just want to lose weight. Some have gluten or dairy intolerances and find that this diet just works better, while others might not have any food allergies but find that a cleaner diet simply feels better.

If you haven't started eating Paleo yet, here are some tips for a successful first few weeks:

1. Get rid of any non-Paleo foods in your pantry or fridge. (You can donate nonperishable items to your local food bank.) Don't keep any cheat items as treats—you'll do so much better if you go all in at the beginning.

2. Stock up on the basics—this book you're holding has everything you need for great meal ideas. Take a look at the Table of Contents (page 7) to get an idea of The Big 15, and then go out and buy eggs, good-quality meats, and lots of vegetables.

3. Plan ahead. Don't leave the house without a healthy snack.

4. Be patient. The first week is the hardest, and you need to give it a good month before you can make any meaningful judgments about your new diet. Drink lots of water, get enough sleep, and take care of yourself. If you do slip up, don't give up—just make a better choice the next time. Every meal or snack is an opportunity to give your body something good, so don't throw in the towel over one cheat meal.

Once you've emptied your pantry and stocked your fridge, you're ready to start!

PANTRY BASICS

Sauces, marinades, and dips can make or break a meal. Being Paleo can be hard when it feels like you can never eat your favorite salad dressing again, or you realize you might have to give up mayonnaise and ketchup. Throughout the book, you'll find condiment recipes like a basic Homemade Mayo (page 47) that you can use on its own or add to for delicious aiolis (think roasted garlic or basil), as well as my favorite vinaigrette recipe (page 89),

which is so easy—you just put all the ingredients in a jar and shake it.

I've also included some dips and marinades like BBQ Sauce (page 131), a Dry Rub (page 229) that's great on most meats but especially ribs, and my mom's Paleo version of Pesto (page 175). You'll notice that these recipes don't have flavor variations, but they're the perfect staples to experiment with your own versions of all of them.

WHY THIS BOOK

Over the years, Paleo has become increasingly mainstream, which is really great—some grocery stores have a Paleo section set up, more restaurants are labeling Paleo-friendly menu items, and some specialty restaurants are even going completely Paleo. But somewhere along the way, this way of eating—or at least the perception of it—became complicated and, often, very expensive. Almond flour can be upwards of $10 a pound, and turning non-Paleo food items like pancakes and muffins into Paleo versions is often a disappointing endeavor, especially if it means later throwing away a significant amount of expensive grain-free supplies.

So for this cookbook, we wanted to return to the basics: real food that's really delicious. You won't find any complicated recipes, and we aren't interested in giving the Paleo treatment to non-Paleo foods like muffins or desserts. We're focused on real food and the ingredients that will make it easy for you to put a meal together in a variety of ways, with plenty of options.

This will be your handbook of go-to Paleo recipes: no-fuss choices to keep you satisfied every day. Changing your diet can be hard at first, so it's really important to keep things simple in the kitchen, making solid meals that taste amazing and don't leave you feeling like you're missing out on bread, rice, or potatoes. And we don't ask you to go and buy expensive grain-free flours or specialty ingredients, either, with the exception of almond flour, which you can just as easily make at home (see the Prep Tip on page 140). All the recipes in this book are straightforward and made with wholesome meats and vegetables that you can find in your local stores.

This book has fifteen chapters based on main ingredients—the Paleo basics, if you will. These include eggs, chicken, beef, pork, seafood, and a variety of vegetables you'll often find in Paleo recipes (like kale, Brussels sprouts, and sweet potatoes). *The Big 15 Cookbook* mission is to provide you with over 150 recipes that are well rounded, easy, and delectable, so you'll never have to wonder what to cook. Each recipe has a couple of variations to give you even more options, and a lot of the dishes can be paired to create larger meals based on whatever ingredients you already have on hand. We've also included labels for the recipes that are dairy-free, nut-free, vegan, and can be made in 30 minutes or less. No expensive shopping trips, no recipes that don't work out in the end, just solid meals you'll enjoy time and time again.

THE YES AND NO LISTS

Going Paleo can sound intimidating because, at first glance, there seem to be a lot of rules, and they're almost all negative. No sugar, no bread, no rice, no dairy . . . before you know it, it feels like you've gutted the entire food pyramid. We focus on the positive side—the foods that you *can* eat on a Paleo diet—but we've included clear "yes" and "no" lists as a guide to the basics.

YES

- Avocados
- Coconut oil
- Eggs
- Fruits
- Grass-fed butter and ghee
- Meats
- Nuts
- Olive oil
- Olives
- Vegetables

NO

- Beans
- Dairy (with the exception of grass-fed butter and ghee)
- Grains
- Legumes (including peanuts)
- Sugar
- White Potatoes

Many people enjoy experimenting with the Paleo diet and seeing which foods work for them, but for the purposes of this book and in the interest of starting your Paleo diet on the right foot, we won't be using any items from the "no" list.

Note: Honey and maple syrup aren't Whole 30-compliant, so if you're doing a program like that, you may want to skip any recipes containing those ingredients for now.

GO-TO PANTRY ITEMS

Paleo cooking can get boring if you don't have enough flavor variations to keep things interesting. To avoid this trap, I recommend keeping a variety of spices in your Paleo pantry. With just a few, you can turn what would otherwise be plain grilled chicken into a delicious chicken curry one night and succulent lemon herb-roasted chicken another.

A note on salt: I like to use kosher salt. I like the texture of it, and I've always used it because that's what my mom uses at home, so I feel very familiar with how much I need in any situation. But you don't need to go out and buy it if you don't already have it. Any salt will do.

Here's a list of the most frequently used herbs and spices you'll find in this book:

- Bay leaves (dried)
- Cayenne pepper (ground)
- Curry powder
- Dill (dried)
- Garlic powder
- Mustard (dried)
- Onion powder
- Oregano (dried)
- Red pepper flakes
- Thyme (dried)

WHY THESE FOODS

The structure of this book is based on the "Paleo Staples;" in other words, the meats and vegetables that you most often find in this style of cooking. These foods merit their own chapters because each one is a building block of a solid Paleo diet.

The proteins (eggs, chicken, beef, pork, fish, and shrimp) do really well with a variety of cooking methods, while the vegetables are versatile and make wonderful main courses as well as side dishes. The proteins and vegetables that make up the chapters in this book are lovely neutral foods that shine no matter the variety of flavor or cooking style you apply to them.

And don't worry; there's no need to go out and buy special equipment or cookware such as a slow cooker or a Dutch oven if you don't have one. You should be able to make all of these recipes with the cooking tools you already have in your kitchen.

OF COCONUTS & OILS

Coconut has become the golden child of the Paleo diet (and every diet, it seems). This fatty, popular food can be added to everything from your coffee, beauty products, or juices to unexpected places like your scrambled eggs or chili. The most common forms of coconut for cooking are coconut oil, coconut flour, and coconut milk. Almost all forms of coconut have incredible health benefits.

A note about butter: Some of the recipes in this book call for grass-fed butter, which is easy to find in good grocery stores and is much better quality than regular butter from grain-fed cows. Other recipes call for ghee, which is clarified butter, meaning that the milk and solids have been removed, leaving only the fat. If you are staying away from dairy completely, feel free to swap butter or ghee for coconut or olive oil. Ghee, coconut oil, and extra-virgin olive oil can all be found in good grocery stores.

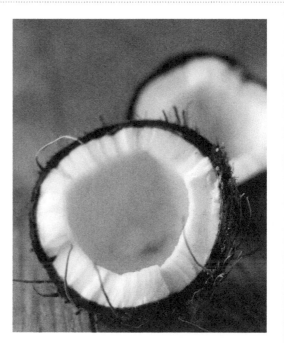

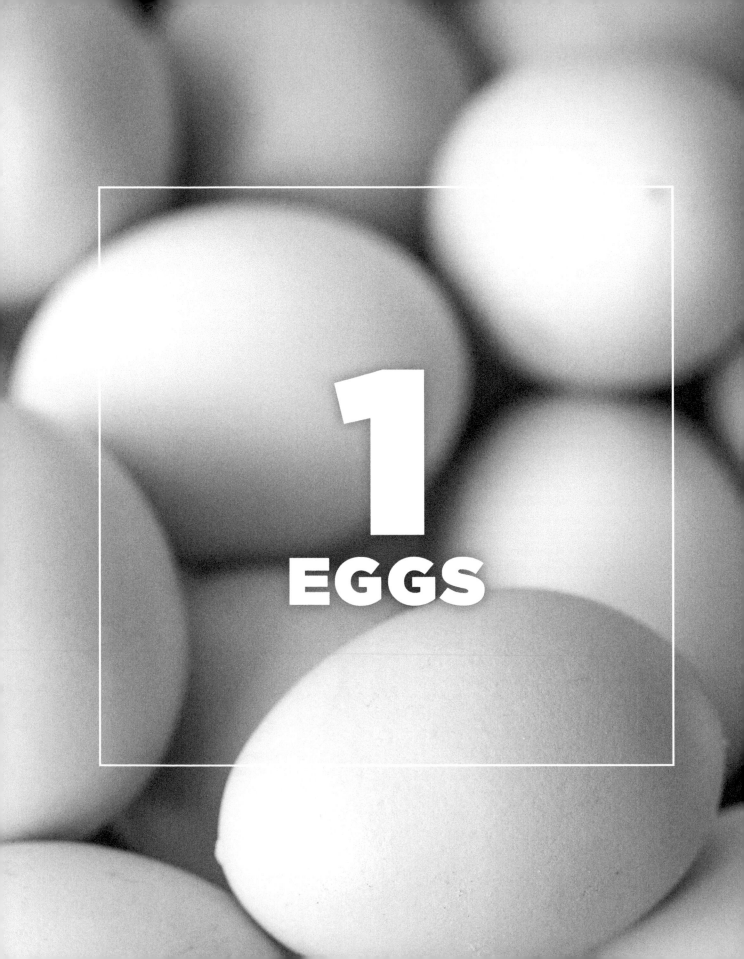

1
EGGS

Whenever people ask me what you can eat on the Paleo diet, my list always starts with eggs. I eat eggs for breakfast almost every day—I usually just quickly scramble them because my husband isn't a big fan of fried eggs. I'll even occasionally have them for lunch (over-medium on top of a big bowl of greens) if I haven't been grocery shopping in a while.

You can do so much with an egg, and these recipes will help you stay creative and switch it up a lot, meaning you'll never get bored. Try one of my favorites—Eggs Benedict (page 25)—which I always make for a crowd, or some of the plan-ahead recipes that will ease your week if you make them on Sunday evenings, like the Egg Muffins (page 27) or Breakfast Casserole (page 29). One of the easiest (and cheapest) proteins out there, eggs are a natural starting point.

BAKED EGGS IN TOMATO SAUCE

I'm a huge fan of baked eggs. Something about them feels incredibly luxurious, which is why I didn't start making them at home until recently. What I now love even more about them is how simple they can be to make, and they're easy to prepare for a crowd if you have guests over. I love the thought of a bunch of friends catching up in the kitchen with coffee as something delicious bakes in the oven for breakfast. It's so cozy. **SERVES 4 TO 6**

PREP TIME: 5 minutes
COOK TIME: 25 minutes

1 tablespoon extra-virgin olive oil

1 small white onion, chopped

2 garlic cloves, minced

1 (16-ounce) can diced tomatoes, drained

1 teaspoon ground paprika

½ to 1 teaspoon red pepper flakes

Salt

Freshly ground black pepper

6 eggs

Chopped fresh basil or parsley, for garnish

1. Preheat the oven to 375°F.

2. In a small saucepan over medium heat, heat the olive oil. Sauté the onion and garlic until the onion is slightly translucent, about 5 minutes.

3. Add the tomatoes, paprika, and red pepper flakes, and give it a stir. Season with salt and pepper, and bring to a low boil. Reduce the heat to low, and simmer for 10 minutes.

4. Transfer the sauce to an ovenproof skillet, and create six small wells in the sauce.

5. Crack 1 egg into each well, put the skillet into the oven, and bake for 7 to 10 minutes, or until the eggs are set.

6. Serve garnished with basil.

VARIATION 1 **SAUSAGE-BAKED EGGS:** For a meatier breakfast, sauté about 1 pound spicy sausage with the garlic and onions before adding the rest of the ingredients and continuing with the recipe as written (shown, right).

VARIATION 2 **BAKED EGGS WITH GREENS:** Prepare the baked eggs in individual ramekins, and serve on a plate with a big salad for lunch.

PREP TIP: This recipe includes directions for making your own tomato sauce, but if you are short on time, a canned marinara sauce will do just fine (as long as it's free of sugar and non-Paleo preservatives; Trader Joe's has a great one in a big green can).

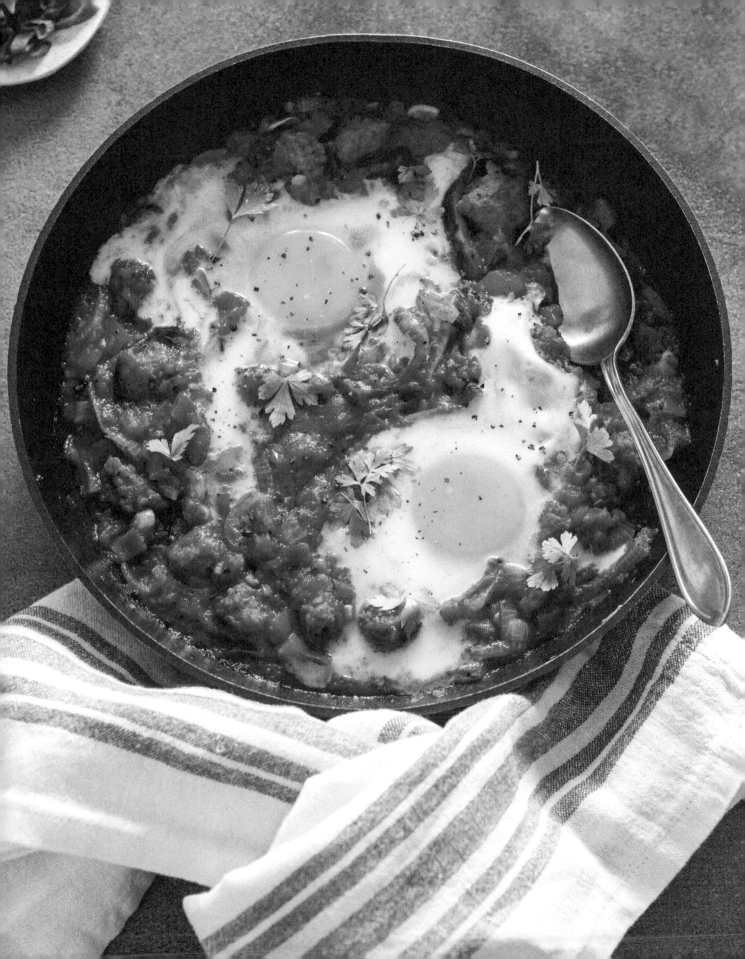

SOUTHWESTERN OMELET

An omelet is definitely one of the more classic breakfast dishes you can make—it's simple and delicious. I like mine on the thinner side so I can fold it completely around the filling. Topped with fresh herbs or a little diced avocado, this Southwestern omelet would make a great lunch or snack as well as the more usual breakfast. **SERVES 1**

PREP TIME: 10 minutes
COOK TIME: 10 minutes

1 tablespoon extra-virgin olive oil or grass-fed butter

¼ red onion, diced

½ garlic clove, minced

1 tablespoon chopped red or green bell pepper (or a mixture)

2 thin slices ham, diced

1 tablespoon chopped fresh tomato

2 eggs

Salt

Freshly ground black pepper

¼ avocado, diced

1 to 2 tablespoons salsa

1. In a large skillet over medium heat, heat the olive oil. Sauté the onion and garlic until the onion is slightly translucent, about 5 minutes.

2. Add the bell pepper, ham, and tomato, and cook for another 2 or 3 minutes, until the ham begins to brown. Remove the mixture from the pan, and set aside. Return the pan to the heat.

3. In a small bowl, whisk the eggs until combined. Pour them into the hot pan, and move the pan around so the egg spreads out evenly across the hot surface. Allow the eggs to set, about 2 minutes, and use a spatula to flip the omelet over.

4. Add the vegetable-ham mixture to the middle of the omelet, spreading it into a broad stripe down the center. Season with salt and pepper, and use a spatula to fold the sides of the omelet over the filling.

5. Transfer the omelet to a plate, top with the avocado and salsa, and serve.

VARIATION 1 **CLASSIC VEGGIE OMELET:** Go vegetarian by replacing the ham with 2 tablespoons Perfect Sautéed Mushrooms (page 207).

VARIATION 2 **CRAB AND ASPARAGUS OMELET:** Sauté 4 or 5 stalks chopped asparagus over medium heat in ½ tablespoon olive oil for 8 to 10 minutes, and then remove from the skillet. Make the omelet as directed in step 3, and fill it with ½ can crabmeat plus the cooked asparagus.

PREP TIP: If you're ever cooking something that requires only egg whites, save the yolks in a container and add them to your next omelet! The same goes for recipes that call for yolks—you can easily add the leftover whites to your breakfast and not have to throw them away.

EGGS BENEDICT

If I'm out to brunch somewhere, then I'm most likely ordering the eggs Benedict. It's delicious and kind of fancy, and it's one of my favorite breakfast dishes. When I was younger, on Christmas morning and other special occasions, my family made our own version of the Egg McMuffin—an English muffin toasted with butter and topped with Canadian bacon, a fried egg, and some cheese. Now that we eat Paleo, we make this version, which takes a little longer but is just as luxuriously creamy and satisfying as the original. **SERVES 4**

PREP TIME: 15 minutes
COOK TIME: 30 minutes

NF

FOR THE MUSHROOMS AND EGGS

8 portobello mushroom caps

2 tablespoons extra-virgin olive oil

Salt

Freshly ground black pepper

Splash white vinegar

8 eggs

4 slices Canadian bacon or thick-cut ham

FOR THE HOLLANDAISE SAUCE

4 egg yolks

1 tablespoon freshly squeezed lemon juice

½ cup (1 stick) unsalted, grass-fed butter, melted

¼ teaspoon ground cayenne pepper

Pinch salt

TO MAKE THE MUSHROOMS AND EGGS

1. Heat a grill pan or large skillet over medium-high heat. Brush both sides of each portobello mushroom cap with olive oil, and season with salt and pepper. Place them in the pan, and cook for 7 to 8 minutes on each side. Remove them from the heat, and set aside.

2. Bring a large saucepan of water to a low simmer. Add the white vinegar. Crack 1 egg into a small dish. Use a large spoon to swirl the water into a slow whirlpool. Carefully slide the egg into the water and, without hitting the egg, continue the swirling motion with the spoon. Allow the egg to cook for a minute or two, until the white has set. Carefully scoop the egg out and place it on a paper towel–lined plate. Repeat with the remaining eggs.

3. In the skillet you used for the mushrooms, heat the Canadian bacon over low heat, about 2 minutes per side.

TO MAKE THE HOLLANDAISE SAUCE

1. Place a heatproof bowl over a pot of simmering water (don't let the bowl actually touch the water).

2. Put the egg yolks and lemon juice in the bowl, and quickly whisk them together until the mixture becomes frothy and starts to expand, about 2 minutes. Slowly drizzle the melted butter in while stirring, and continue to whisk until the sauce has doubled in size, 5 to 6 minutes. Remove from the heat, and add the cayenne and salt.

3. Serve immediately or keep warm until ready to serve. ›

TO ASSEMBLE THE EGGS BENEDICT

Plate each portobello mushroom cap with the bottom side facing up. Add a slice of Canadian bacon to each, top each piece of bacon with a poached egg and some hollandaise sauce, and serve.

VARIATION 1 **SOUTHWESTERN BENEDICT:** Switch out the Canadian bacon for ¼ cup Pulled Pork (page 74) or beef brisket and add a teaspoon of chipotle seasoning to your hollandaise for a spicier, heftier dish.

VARIATION 2 **TOMATO BENEDICT:** Use thick slices of tomato instead of the portobello mushrooms if you're short on time and want to skip a step. This is how I order eggs Benedict in a restaurant.

PREP TIP: Poaching eggs can take some practice, but you can find egg-poaching gadgets out there that make it a lot easier. You can also make the eggs first and keep them in a very low heat oven (200°F or lower) until you've assembled the rest of the dish; just undercook them a tiny bit in the pan so you don't overcook them in the oven.

EGG MUFFINS

Egg muffins are the ultimate Sunday meal prep recipe. I often visit Richmond, Virginia, to spend the weekend at my friend Tina's house, and I'm always so impressed by how organized she is when it comes to getting ready for the week. We stood in the kitchen together with coffee and started to make breakfast for everyone, and as we started assembling a Spicy Sausage Frittata (page 33), she grabbed extra veggies and tossed them into a bowl to become egg muffins that would get her and her husband through a busy week of breakfasts. Eating well takes planning, but only a little. **SERVES 6**

PREP TIME: 10 minutes
COOK TIME: 40 minutes

1 tablespoon extra-virgin olive oil, plus extra for greasing

1 red onion, finely diced

2 garlic cloves, minced

10 ounces mushrooms, sliced

1 green bell pepper, finely diced

12 eggs

12 slices bacon

1. Preheat the oven to 350°F.

2. In a large skillet over medium heat, heat the olive oil. Sauté the onion and garlic until the onion is slightly translucent, about 5 minutes. Add the mushrooms, and cook for another 5 to 10 minutes. Stir in the bell pepper. Remove the skillet from the heat.

3. In a medium bowl, whisk the eggs together. Set aside.

4. Lightly grease a 12-cup muffin tin with olive oil. Carefully wrap a strip of bacon around the inside of each muffin well.

5. Pour some of the egg mixture into each bacon-lined muffin well, and then spoon the sautéed veggie mixture into each one.

6. Bake for 25 minutes, or until the eggs are firm, and serve.

VARIATION 1 **VEGGIE EGG MUFFINS:** Skip the bacon and pour the egg muffin "batter" right into the greased muffin tins. They'll pop right out.

VARIATION 2 **SAUSAGE AND EGG MUFFINS:** Cook 10 ounces spicy Italian sausage or just regular breakfast sausage, and let it cool. Add it to the egg mixture, and continue with the recipe as written.

PREP TIP: Cutting up all your veggies as soon as you bring them home from the store is a fantastic way to make sure they're always ready to go into any recipe. I've found that it really helps us reduce our food waste as well.

EGG SALAD

Egg salad may seem like a dish best served with bread, but once you've been Paleo for a while, you start to find new and easier ways to enjoy the spread-ier types of meals out there. This comforting salad, with its mustard and pickle tang, is wonderful wrapped in a big leaf of lettuce or dipped into with celery sticks. My favorite way to enjoy egg salad, however, is scooped onto a huge bowl of field greens with a little bit of Balsamic Vinaigrette (page 89). **SERVES 4**

PREP TIME: 5 minutes
COOK TIME: 10 minutes

8 eggs

½ cup Homemade Mayo (page 47)

1 teaspoon yellow mustard

1 tablespoon dill pickle relish

Salt

Freshly ground black pepper

1 or 2 tablespoons sliced scallions, for garnish

1. Place the eggs in a large saucepan with enough water to cover them. Bring the water to a boil, and boil for 10 minutes. Use a large spoon to transfer the eggs to a colander, and place under running cold water to cool. Peel and set aside until ready to make the salad.

2. In a large bowl, mash the eggs carefully. Add the Homemade Mayo, mustard, and relish, and stir until well incorporated. Season with salt and pepper.

3. Serve topped with a sprinkle of scallions.

VARIATION 1 **EGG SALAD IN BACON BOWLS:** Turn a muffin tin upside down, and cover the outside of each well with a slice of bacon. Bake at 400°F for about 10 minutes, or until the bacon is crispy. Remove the tin from the oven, cool, remove the bacon cups, and scoop egg salad into the cups.

VARIATION 2 **NIÇOISE EGG SALAD:** Mix the hardboiled eggs with a 5-ounce can tuna, 1 tablespoon finely chopped red onion, ¼ cup chopped cherry tomatoes, and ½ cup chopped cooked green beans. Serve over field greens or romaine lettuce.

PREP TIP: Every Sunday night I like to hard-boil a whole dozen eggs. I can eat them by themselves, add them to salads, or quickly whip up some egg salad. Add this to your weekly meal prep, and you'll never have to think too hard about breakfast!

BREAKFAST CASSEROLE

Having a go-to breakfast casserole recipe can be a lifesaver for brunch parties or when hosting overnight guests. It takes a little planning, but you can do the majority of the work ahead of time and just cook it in the morning. I love the thought of sneaking down to the kitchen while everyone is still asleep and popping a big baking dish of hearty goodness into the oven so guests wake up to the smell of breakfast waiting for them. **SERVES 8 TO 10**

PREP TIME: 10 minutes
COOK TIME: 1 hour, 40 minutes

3 tablespoons extra-virgin olive oil, divided

¼ onion, chopped (2 to 3 tablespoons)

1 garlic clove, minced

1 large sweet potato, diced

8 ounces mushrooms, sliced

Salt

Freshly ground black pepper

10 ounces breakfast sausage

10 eggs

2 tablespoons sliced scallion, for garnish

1. Preheat the oven to 350°F.

2. In a large skillet over medium heat, heat 1½ tablespoons of olive oil. Sauté the onion and garlic until the onion is slightly translucent, about 5 minutes. Add the sweet potato, and cook until fork-tender, about another 15 minutes. Spoon the mixture into an 8-by-12-inch baking dish.

3. Add the remaining 1½ tablespoons of olive oil to the skillet, and sauté the mushrooms until browned, 5 to 7 minutes. Season with salt and pepper, and add them to the baking dish as a second layer.

4. Add the sausage to the skillet, and cook until no more pink remains, 7 to 10 minutes. Season with salt and pepper, and add to the baking dish as a third layer.

5. In a large bowl, whisk the eggs well, season with salt and pepper, and pour over the casserole mixture in the baking dish. Bake for about 1 hour, or until the eggs are no longer runny.

6. Serve hot, garnished with a sprinkle of sliced scallion.

VARIATION 1 **BLT CASSEROLE:** Replace the sausage with bacon, and serve the casserole topped with ½ cup chopped lettuce and a side of Ranch Dressing (page 75).

VARIATION 2 **PIZZA CASSEROLE:** For meat lovers, skip the sweet potato and add 6 ounces sliced pepperoni to the casserole dish. Serve with a side of warm (sugar-free) pizza sauce.

PREP TIP: Assemble the casserole up to the end of step 4 ahead of time, and refrigerate until ready to bake. Add the eggs and bake the morning you plan to serve the casserole.

DEVILED EGGS

Deviled eggs are a fun little party dish that I love to serve as an appetizer anytime I have people over. They also double as a great snack or quick breakfast, so I tend to make a lot of them at a time. They have a charming, almost vintage vibe that I find entertaining, and they're surprisingly easy to add to so you never get bored with them. **SERVES 6**

PREP TIME: 20 minutes
COOK TIME: 10 minutes

6 eggs

½ cup Homemade Mayo (page 47)

1 tablespoon finely chopped red onion

½ teaspoon dried mustard

½ teaspoon dill pickle relish

½ teaspoon white vinegar

Salt

Freshly ground black pepper

Paprika, for garnish

1. Hard-boil the eggs by placing them in a saucepan with enough water to cover them. Bring the water to a boil, and boil for 10 minutes. Use a large spoon to transfer the eggs to a colander, and place under cold running water to cool. Peel and set aside until ready to make the rest of the dish.

2. Halve each egg lengthwise, and pop the yolks out into a large bowl. Add the Homemade Mayo, onion, mustard, relish, and vinegar, and mix until smooth. Season with salt and pepper.

3. Spoon the yolk mixture into a piping bag (or just use a large resealable plastic bag and cut one corner off). Carefully fill each egg white half with the yolk filling.

4. Sprinkle with paprika and serve.

VARIATION 1 **SMOKED SALMON DEVILED EGGS:** Top each deviled egg with a slice of smoked salmon, a couple of capers, and ½ teaspoon finely chopped red onion.

VARIATION 2 **SHRIMP DEVILED EGGS:** Mix the deviled egg filling with 1 teaspoon minced fresh parsley, 1 teaspoon minced fresh dill, and 2 to 3 ounces chopped cooked shrimp.

PALEO PAIR: Serve alongside Kale Salad with Onion and Avocado (page 128) or Shaved Brussels Sprout Salad with Apple Cider Vinaigrette (page 179).

EGGS AND SOLDIERS

I've been enamored with soft-boiled eggs since I read Molly Wizenberg's romantic piece on Saveur.com titled "The Seven-Minute Egg." These eggs are even quicker, because you want a runny yolk to dip the Paleo "soldiers" into. These are usually strips of toast, but in our case, they're sweet and salty bacon-wrapped sweet potato wedges. This recipe is unique and a little fancy, but perfect for adults and children alike. **SERVES 4**

PREP TIME: 10 minutes
COOK TIME: 45 minutes

2 sweet potatoes, each cut into about 8 (¼-inch) wedges

8 slices bacon, halved

8 eggs

1. Preheat the oven to 400°F.

2. Wrap each sweet potato wedge with ½ piece of bacon. Place on a baking sheet, and bake for 30 to 40 minutes, turning the potatoes over halfway through the cooking time. Remove from the oven, and let cool slightly.

3. Toward the end of the baking time, bring a medium saucepan of water to a boil. Using a spoon, carefully lower the eggs into the boiling water, and cook for 6 minutes. Use a spoon to transfer the eggs to a colander, and run them under cold water to stop further cooking. Place into egg cups, and cut off the tops.

4. Serve 2 eggs and 4 potato wedges per person. To eat, dip the bacon-wrapped sweet potatoes into the egg yolk. When you've eaten the sweet potatoes, spoon out the rest of the eggs onto your plate.

VARIATION 1 **AVOCADO SOLDIERS:** Instead of quartered sweet potatoes, wrap quartered avocado in halved slices of bacon. You can cook these for a few minutes on each side in a skillet instead of in the oven since the avocado doesn't really need to bake.

VARIATION 2 **ASPARAGUS SOLDIERS:** Use asparagus instead of sweet potatoes if you would like more green vegetables with your breakfast—just snap the ends off the asparagus stalks and drizzle with about a tablespoon of olive oil, then roast at 425°F for 15 to 20 minutes.

PALEO PAIR: For a light lunch, serve the Eggs and Soldiers over 1 or 2 cups field greens.

EGG SCRAMBLE WITH VEGGIES

My husband and I have this for breakfast at least twice a week—it's a super simple breakfast that makes it really easy to get rid of leftover veggies. A little onion, some garlic, and whatever vegetables and meat you need to get rid of, this breakfast can be different every time, but the basic recipe is always the same. It only takes about 20 minutes, which makes it a great weekday breakfast even when you're busy. **SERVES 3 TO 4**

PREP TIME: 5 minutes
COOK TIME: 20 minutes

2 tablespoons extra-virgin olive oil or grass-fed butter

½ onion, finely diced

10 ounces mushrooms, sliced

2 small zucchini, finely diced

1 green or red bell pepper, finely diced

2 garlic cloves, minced

5 or 6 eggs

Salt

Freshly ground black pepper

1. In a large skillet over medium heat, heat the olive oil. Sauté the onion until slightly translucent, about 5 minutes. Add the mushrooms, and cook for 5 minutes more. Finally, throw in the zucchini, bell pepper, and garlic. Increase the heat to medium-high, and cook for 5 more minutes.

2. In a medium bowl, whisk the eggs together, and season with salt and pepper. Move the veggies to one side of the pan, and add the eggs to the other side. Quickly scramble them, and begin incorporating the vegetables into the eggs. Lower the heat and cook until the eggs are no longer runny, about another 5 minutes.

3. Serve immediately.

VARIATION 1 **AVOCADO SALSA SCRAMBLE:** Serve this recipe topped with 2 tablespoons salsa and half a diced avocado.

VARIATION 2 **MEAT LOVER'S SCRAMBLE:** Cook ½ pound sausage or ham with the eggs, either with or without the veggies listed above.

PREP TIP: You can customize this recipe any way you want; if you have any veggies or meat at all left over in your fridge, give them a try! Find your favorite combinations, and keep experimenting.

SPICY SAUSAGE FRITTATA

Frittatas are beautiful and make a great breakfast or lunch. I love how easily you can customize them, using whatever veggies and meat are left in your refrigerator on a Sunday morning without it ever feeling like a meal thrown together with leftovers. We start the frittata on the stove to get a crunchy outside and then transfer it to the oven to bake off, almost like a soufflé. It's easy and delicious, and it all happens in one pan, which makes for easy cleanup. **SERVES 6 TO 8**

PREP TIME: 10 minutes
COOK TIME: 30 minutes

DF **NF**

1 tablespoon extra-virgin olive oil

1 red onion, finely diced

1 or 2 garlic cloves, minced

1 green or red bell pepper, finely diced

8 eggs

10 ounces spicy Italian sausage, cooked

1 cup cherry tomatoes

Salt

Freshly ground black pepper

1. Preheat the oven to 350°F.

2. In a large ovenproof skillet over medium heat, heat the olive oil. Sauté the onion, garlic, and bell pepper until the onion is slightly translucent, about 5 minutes.

3. In a large bowl, gently whisk the eggs together until just combined. Stir in the sautéed veggies, sausage, and tomatoes. Season with salt and pepper.

4. Pour the egg mixture into the skillet, and allow it to cook until the edges begin to pull away, 3 to 5 minutes.

5. Transfer the skillet to the oven, and cook until the frittata is set, 15 to 20 minutes.

6. Serve immediately.

VARIATION 1 **COBB FRITTATA:** For a less spicy dish, omit the sausage and peppers, and replace them with 10 ounces diced chicken; then top the frittata with a sliced avocado.

VARIATION 2 **SMOKED SALMON FRITTATA:** Replace the meat and peppers with asparagus, and top the cooked frittata with about 6 ounces smoked salmon and a handful of sliced scallions.

PREP TIP: Make a really large frittata, cut it up, and freeze it for later. Defrost overnight in the refrigerator, and reheat in the oven before serving.

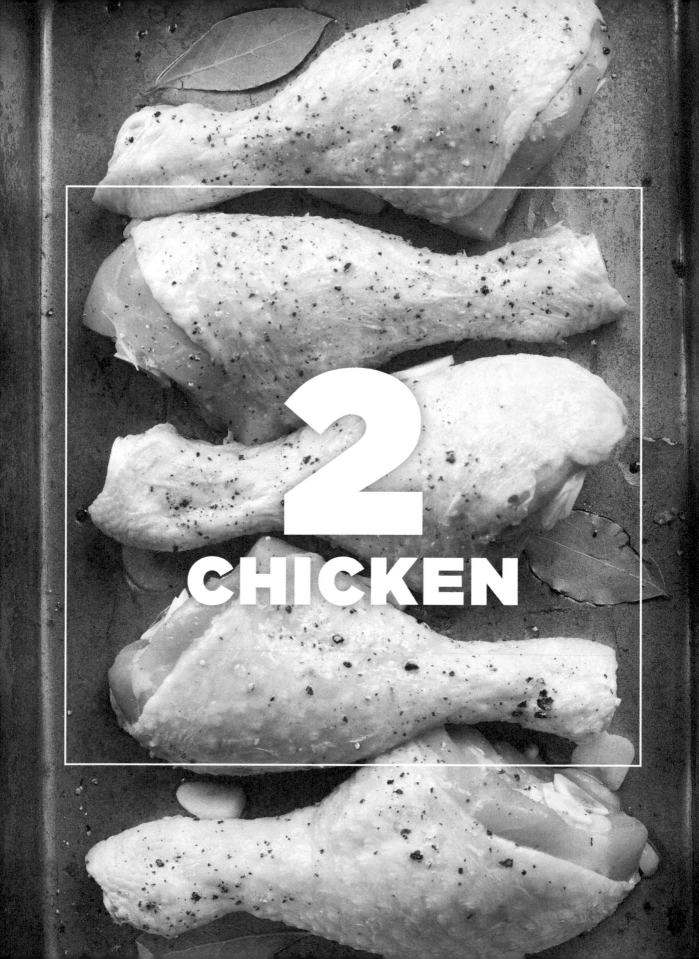

2
CHICKEN

Oh, chicken—probably the most used meat out there, at least for my family. Every week I load up at the market with one whole chicken for roasting and bone broth, a few breasts, lots of thighs (they're my favorite because they're more flavorful, and I find them really hard to overcook, which is not the case with breasts), and sometimes a package of legs. I'm also a big fan of canned chicken (although you can very easily boil a few breasts and then shred or dice them) for chicken salad.

This chapter is full of recipes for using the different parts of the chicken, from legs to breasts to my weekly roast chicken ritual. I include a bone broth recipe for soup, because I love a warm mug of broth when I'm feeling under the weather or just want a light snack. You can read a lot more about bone broth and all of its health benefits online, but it's super easy to make and is a great base for any kind of soup.

A few of the recipes in this chapter are family recipes that I'm so happy to be sharing with you, like my mom's Chicken Piccata (page 43), and I hope some of them will become your new favorite meals.

CHICKEN SOUP

If you've done any reading on Paleo, I'm sure you've encountered some discussion about bone broth, which is basically just a very concentrated, oftentimes homemade, stock. It has myriad health benefits and is absolutely delicious, which is why I roast chickens so often, so I can make bone broth afterward. This chicken soup starts with homemade bone broth, and then we add vegetables and more chicken. It's tasty and comforting and doesn't take too long, especially if you have the broth ready beforehand. **SERVES 8 TO 10**

PREP TIME: 5 minutes
COOK TIME: 3 to 12 hours

Carcass and drippings from Roasted Lemon Chicken (page 40)

1½ onions, quartered, divided

3 carrots, chopped, divided

2 garlic cloves, smashed

2 zucchini, diced or spiralized into noodles

10 to 12 ounces diced cooked chicken breast or thighs

1. In a Dutch oven or large stockpot over medium-high heat, combine the chicken carcass and drippings, 1 onion, 2 carrots, the garlic, and enough water to cover the chicken carcass by 2 or more inches, and bring to a boil.

2. Reduce the heat to low, cover, and simmer for at least 3 hours, and up to 12 hours.

3. Strain the broth through a sieve into a large pan. Discard the chicken carcass and soggy vegetables.

4. In the same Dutch oven over medium heat, sauté the remaining half onion and 1 remaining carrot with the zucchini for about 5 minutes. Add the cooked chicken, and pour the broth on top.

5. Simmer over low heat until ready to serve.

VARIATION 1 **SLOW COOKER BONE BROTH:** Add the chicken carcass, onion, carrots, and garlic to a slow cooker, and cover with water. Cook on low for 12 hours, and strain.

VARIATION 2 **EGG-DROP SOUP:** For an extra boost of protein without adding meat, bring 1½ cups bone broth to a boil. In a small bowl, whisk 1 egg together with a pinch of salt. Once the broth is boiling, turn off the heat and slowly pour the egg into the soup while stirring. Garnish with sliced scallions, and serve immediately.

PREP TIP: Make an extra batch of broth and freeze it in an ice cube tray so you'll have it ready for other meals or to defrost and drink as a snack. On the other hand, if you want to make soup but don't have time to cook the broth, store-bought will work in a pinch.

FAJITA-STUFFED CHICKEN BREAST

My go-to order at a Mexican restaurant is fajitas. They don't come loaded with cheese, and it's easy enough to skip the rice, beans, and tortillas to keep it Paleo. For this recipe I wanted to make an easy weeknight dish that would satisfy your cravings for Mexican takeout. When cravings hit after a long day, it can be hard to stick to Paleo. This fajita-stuffed chicken breast should do the trick. **SERVES 4**

PREP TIME: 10 minutes
COOK TIME: 30 minutes

NF

4 tablespoons grass-fed butter, divided

1 onion, sliced

2 garlic cloves, minced

1 green bell pepper, cut into strips

1 red bell pepper, cut into strips

1 yellow bell pepper, cut into strips

2 tablespoons taco seasoning

Salt

Freshly ground black pepper

1 pound boneless skinless chicken breasts

1. In a large pan over medium heat, melt 2 tablespoons of butter. Sauté the onion and garlic until the onion is slightly translucent, about 5 minutes. Add the green, red, and yellow peppers, and continue to cook until everything is caramelized, about 10 minutes more.

2. Remove the veggies from the heat, and set them aside in a medium bowl. Stir in the taco seasoning, and season with salt and pepper.

3. Using a sharp knife, slice a pocket in the side of each chicken breast. Spoon about 2 tablespoons of the fajita vegetable mixture into each piece of chicken. Season the outside of the chicken breasts with salt and pepper.

4. In the same pan over medium heat, heat the remaining 2 tablespoons of butter. Cook the chicken for about 7 minutes on each side, or until golden and cooked all the way through.

5. Serve immediately.

VARIATION 1 **SPINACH ARTICHOKE–STUFFED CHICKEN:** If you're not crazy about peppers, skip them and make the filling with 1 cup sautéed spinach and 1 can chopped artichokes.

VARIATION 2 **GUACAMOLE-STUFFED CHICKEN:** In a large bowl, smash and mix 2 ripe avocados with 1 crushed garlic clove and a splash of hot sauce. Add the juice of half a lime and ½ tablespoon chopped fresh cilantro. Stuff the chicken with the guacamole in step 3, and continue with the recipe as written. Garnish with wedges of lime before serving.

PREP TIP: Assemble the dish ahead of time so when you're ready for dinner, you can just throw it in a pan and cook.

CHICKEN SALAD

Chicken salad is an absolute go-to Paleo lunch when I'm busy. Sometimes I'll order it if I'm out, but most of the time I like to make it myself. You can easily add almost any flavor or spice to chicken salad, and it's delicious served on top of fresh greens or in a big leaf of lettuce as a wrap. Or you can just eat it by itself with a fork. It's the perfect Paleo staple, whether you're looking for a full meal or just a snack. **SERVES 4**

PREP TIME: 10 minutes
COOK TIME: None

2 (12.5-ounce) cans
chicken breast

¾ to 1 cup Homemade Mayo
(page 47), depending on desired
consistency/creaminess

1 cup grapes, halved

1 celery stalk, diced

1 or 2 scallions, thinly sliced

Salt

Freshly ground black pepper

1. In a large bowl, stir together the chicken, Homemade Mayo, grapes, celery, and scallions until well combined. Season with salt and pepper.

2. Serve immediately or refrigerate until ready to eat.

VARIATION 1 **CHICKEN SALAD WITH APPLES:** Replace the grapes with diced apples for more of a crunch—green or red would work, although I'm partial to red. If you're feeling summery, try diced mango instead.

VARIATION 2 **CURRY CHICKEN SALAD:** Swap out the grapes for ½ cup raisins and add 1½ tablespoons curry powder if you're in the mood for something more piquant.

PREP TIP: Canned chicken is easy to find and even easier to use, but if you have 2 or 3 chicken breasts in your freezer or refrigerator and no idea what to do with them, gently boil them for 15 to 20 minutes. Remove them from the water, allow to cool, and shred with two forks.

CURRY CHICKEN

Curries are often a great Paleo choice when you're out at an Indian or Thai restaurant, because they are straightforward sauces that usually contain coconut milk instead of dairy. I love ordering it when I'm out, but I'm a big fan of making my own even more Paleo-friendly version at home. You can make this recipe a lot hotter if you like things on the spicier side, or you could skip the red pepper flakes altogether if you're in the mood for something mild. **SERVES 4**

PREP TIME: 10 minutes
COOK TIME: 35 minutes

`DF` `NF`

2 tablespoons extra-virgin olive oil

½ onion, sliced

2 garlic cloves, minced

1½ pounds boneless skinless chicken thighs, diced

2 teaspoons curry powder

¼ teaspoon red pepper flakes

¼ teaspoon garlic powder

Salt

Freshly ground black pepper

½ cup chicken broth

½ (13.5-ounce) can full-fat coconut milk

1 to 2 tablespoons sliced scallion

1. In a large skillet over medium heat, heat the olive oil. Sauté the onion and garlic until the onion is slightly translucent, about 5 minutes. Reduce the heat to medium-low, and continue to cook for another 10 minutes.

2. Return the heat to medium, and add the chicken. Cook for 7 to 8 minutes, until golden brown. Add the curry powder, red pepper flakes, and garlic powder, and season with salt and pepper.

3. Pour the chicken broth into the pan, and stir to deglaze, scraping up the browned bits from the bottom. Add the coconut milk while continuing to stir. Cook on low for another 5 to 10 minutes.

4. Serve hot, garnished with the scallions.

`VARIATION 1` **CHICKEN CURRY SOUP:** Make this recipe in a saucepan instead of a skillet, and add 3 to 4 more cups chicken broth. Taste and season with salt, pepper, and perhaps more curry powder. You could also cook the chicken thighs whole in a 300°F oven for about 40 minutes, until browned and cooked through, and shred after cooking for a different texture in the soup.

`VARIATION 2` **SHRIMP CURRY:** Make this recipe with shrimp! Use 1 to 2 pounds peeled and deveined shrimp with the tails removed. They only need to cook for about 5 minutes in step 2, until pink, so dinner will be on the table even faster.

PREP TIP: Dice the chicken ahead of time and store in the fridge or freezer until ready to cook. For some reason, cutting raw chicken is one of my least favorite prep things, and doing it ahead of time always makes dinner so much easier.

ROASTED LEMON CHICKEN

I try to make a roast chicken every weekend—it's a great way to make sure you have leftovers for the week, and I always make bone broth with the carcass (see the Chicken Soup recipe on page 36). For so long, roasting a whole chicken seemed really intimidating, like it was the holy grail of housewives everywhere; but I soon learned there's nothing particularly complicated about it. Once you get the hang of it, the whole thing becomes a nice habit. **SERVES 4**

PREP TIME: 10 minutes
COOK TIME: 1 hour, 40 minutes
TOTAL TIME: 2 hours

1 (5 to 6 pound) chicken

Pinch dried oregano

Pinch red pepper flakes

Pinch celery seed

Pinch dried parsley flakes

Pinch dried sage

Salt

Freshly ground black pepper

1 lemon, halved

1 garlic bulb, cut in half width-wise and outer skin removed, 1 clove reserved

1 dried bay leaf

1 tablespoon extra-virgin olive oil

½ onion, quartered

2 carrots, cut into 1-inch pieces

PALEO PAIR: Serve with Bacon Brussels Sprouts (page 178) for a complete dinner.

1. Preheat the oven to 375°F.

2. Place the chicken on a large plate or a plastic cutting board. Make sure the giblets have been removed from inside the bird, and pat the skin dry with a paper towel.

3. Season the chicken with the oregano, red pepper flakes, celery seed, parsley flakes, and sage, season with salt and pepper, and stuff the inside of the bird with the lemon, garlic bulb, and bay leaf.

4. In a large pan or Dutch oven over medium-high heat, heat the olive oil. Sauté the onion and the reserved garlic clove until translucent while searing the bird breast-side down in the pan to brown the skin, about 5 minutes. Flip the bird over, and transfer it and the onion and garlic to a roasting pan (or leave it in the Dutch oven, if using).

5. Add the carrots, and transfer the pan to the oven. Roast for 1½ hours, or until the juices run clear when the thigh is poked with a knife.

6. Remove the bird from the oven, and allow it to rest for 10 minutes before carving.

7. Keep the drippings, leftover veggies, and chicken carcass to make broth (see page 36).

VARIATION 1 **ROSEMARY-LEMON CHICKEN:** Use fresh oregano instead of dried, and stuff the bird with several fresh rosemary sprigs, reserving a tablespoon or so of the leaves for garnish (shown, right).

VARIATION 2 **CRISPY BUTTER CHICKEN:** Before roasting, slather the bird with plenty of grass-fed butter for an extra-crispy skin. Cut up 1 or 2 tablespoons butter, and stuff it underneath the skin of the breast.

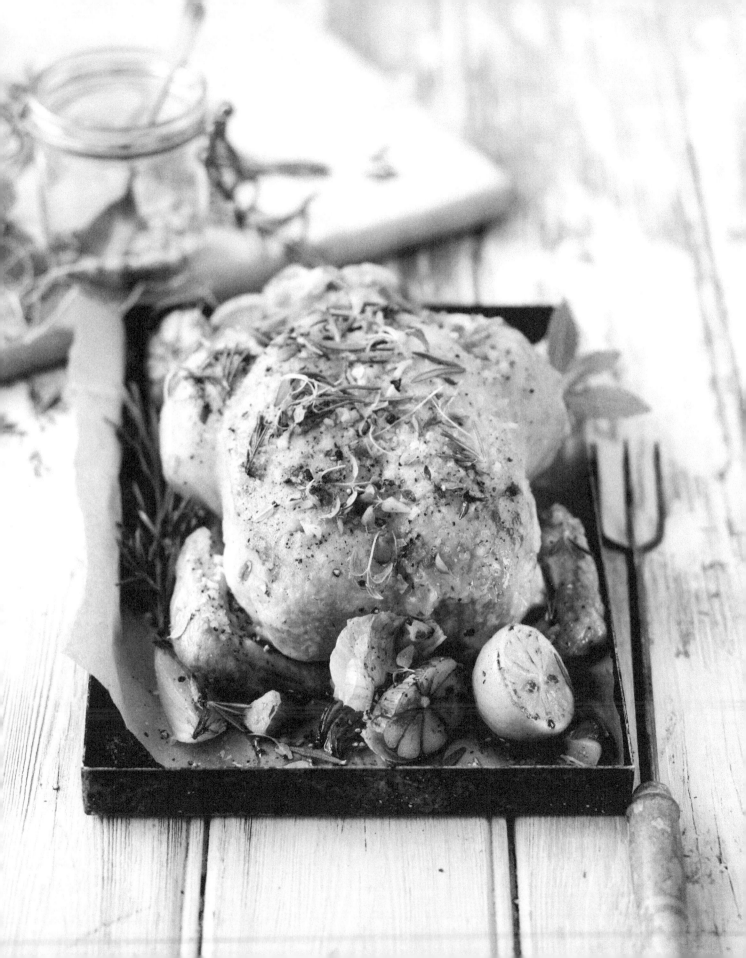

CHICKEN CHILI

My brother and I make this chili together every fall, and it's one of my favorite traditions. Cooking with Sean and coming up with new recipes for our collection is always so exciting. This chili is definitely spicy but not overpowering—if you like it a little milder, you can cut back on the red pepper flakes and/or cayenne. It's great all year round, although I'm partial to it in those first few weekends of autumn when the air is crisp and cool. **SERVES 4 TO 6**

PREP TIME: 15 minutes
COOK TIME: At least 2 hours, 15 minutes

2 tablespoons extra-virgin olive oil

1 large onion, diced

2 or 3 garlic cloves, chopped

1 medium red bell pepper, chopped

1 medium yellow bell pepper, chopped

2 pounds ground chicken

1 (28-ounce) can crushed tomatoes

1½ teaspoons red pepper flakes

1 tablespoon chili powder

1 teaspoon ground cumin

1 teaspoon ground paprika

¾ teaspoon dried mustard

¾ teaspoon ground coriander

½ teaspoon ground allspice

½ teaspoon dried oregano

2 cups chicken broth

½ cup apple cider vinegar

1½ teaspoons ground cayenne pepper, divided

1. In a large cast iron pot over medium heat, heat the olive oil. Sauté the onion, garlic, and red and yellow bell peppers until they have softened, about 5 minutes.

2. Add the chicken, and brown, 5 to 10 minutes, stirring with a wooden spoon to break up the larger pieces.

3. After the chicken is mostly browned, add the tomatoes. Give it all a good stir, and add the red pepper flakes, chili powder, cumin, paprika, mustard, coriander, allspice, and oregano.

4. Bring the chili to a low boil, and reduce the heat to low. Simmer the chili for at least 2 hours. Periodically stir in some chicken broth when it starts getting thick. You may not need the whole 2 cups.

5. About 20 minutes before serving, stir in the apple cider vinegar. Add the cayenne ½ teaspoon at a time, stirring it in and tasting for heat before adding more, until it is as spicy as you like it.

6. Serve immediately.

VARIATION 1 **SLOW COOKER CHICKEN CHILI:** Sauté the onion, garlic, and peppers and brown the chicken as written in the original recipe. Transfer to a slow cooker, and add the remaining ingredients. Cook on low for 8 to 10 hours.

VARIATION 2 **EXTRA-SPICY CHILI:** Garnish with scallions for a little pop of brightness and some pickled jalapeños if you really like it hot.

PREP TIP: If you have the time, start this recipe in the morning and allow it sit on the stove over low heat for as long as possible. The longer it has to cook, the better the flavor will be.

CHICKEN PICCATA

My mom makes this dish all the time, so apart from the fact that it tastes great, I love it because it reminds me of her. Traditional chicken piccata is usually dipped in a flour batter and topped with cheese, but this recipe is simpler, with sautéed chicken and lots of delicious, buttery mushrooms and bright lemon juice. It also scales up easily, so it would be perfect to make for a crowd. **SERVES 2**

PREP TIME: 10 minutes
COOK TIME: 25 minutes

NF

1 pound thinly sliced chicken breast or tenders

Salt

Freshly ground black pepper

1 tablespoon grass-fed butter

1 tablespoon extra-virgin olive oil

1 tablespoon freshly squeezed lemon juice, divided

¼ cup chicken broth, divided

1 tablespoon capers, drained, divided

10 ounces mushrooms, white button or baby bellas, sliced

1. Lay the chicken out on a plastic cutting board, and cover with plastic wrap. Pound the pieces out to get them as thin as possible. Remove the plastic wrap, and season with salt and pepper.

2. In a large skillet over medium heat, heat the butter and olive oil. When it is hot, quickly sauté half the chicken in a single layer until it begins to brown, about 4 minutes on each side. Add half the lemon juice, half the chicken broth, and half the capers. Cover the pan and let cook for 2 minutes more. Transfer the chicken from the pan to a serving dish.

3. Repeat step 2 with the remaining chicken.

4. Finally, sauté the mushrooms in the same pan for about 5 minutes.

5. Pile the cooked mushrooms on top of the chicken, and serve.

VARIATION 1 **PALEO CHICKEN PICCATA WITH ARTICHOKES:** Add a can of artichoke hearts to the mushrooms, and sauté them together.

VARIATION 2 **GREEN BEAN CHICKEN PICCATA:** In a small saucepan, boil about 10 ounces chopped green beans for 4 to 5 minutes. Drain and plunge into a bowl of cold water to stop them cooking. Serve with the chicken piccata.

PALEO PAIR: Serve with zucchini noodles. If you don't have a spiralizing tool or vegetable peeler, just julienne the zucchini with a knife. Quickly sauté the noodles in a teaspoon of hot olive oil, and they're ready to eat!

CHICKEN WITH ROASTED RED PEPPERS AND OLIVES

My mom is always making recipes like this one. She moves about the kitchen swiftly, often with a glass of wine in her hand, and somehow makes magic happen with just a few seemingly random ingredients. She'll pull out the olives at the last minute, as though she had forgotten about them, or maybe only just thought to throw them in. It's this kind of cooking that I love the most— the kind that involves the quick dip of a spoon into the sauce to taste what's missing. It's how family recipes come to be. **SERVES 4**

PREP TIME: 10 minutes
COOK TIME: 20 minutes

30 **NF**

2 tablespoons grass-fed butter

1 onion, sliced

1 garlic clove, minced

1 pound boneless skinless chicken breast, sliced lengthwise into tenders

½ cup white wine or chicken broth

1 can artichoke hearts, drained and chopped

2 or 3 roasted red peppers, diced

⅓ cup Kalamata olives

¼ cup chopped fresh parsley

1. In a large skillet over medium heat, heat the butter. Sauté the onion and garlic until the onion is slightly translucent, about 5 minutes. Add the chicken to the pan, and brown, about 5 minutes more.

2. Deglaze the pan with the wine or broth, stirring to scrape up the browned bits from the bottom, and then add the artichoke hearts and roasted red peppers. Cook for 7 to 10 more minutes.

3. Add the olives during the final minute of cooking, and serve garnished with the parsley.

VARIATION 1 **SPINACH AND MUSHROOM CHICKEN:** Before adding the chicken in step 1, add 1 cup well-washed and drained spinach and 8 to 10 ounces sliced mushrooms to the pan. Sauté for about 10 minutes, and then add the chicken and continue with the recipe as written. Skip the olives.

VARIATION 2 **SUN-DRIED TOMATO CHICKEN WITH ARTICHOKES:** Substitute the roasted red peppers for chopped sun-dried tomatoes for a stronger flavor.

PALEO PAIR: Serve with Roasted Broccoli with Lemon (page 135) for a complete dinner.

PROSCIUTTO-WRAPPED CHICKEN THIGHS

This chicken is incredibly flavorful and easy to make—it's like a fancier Paleo version of chicken cordon bleu, without the cheese or breading. We use prosciutto instead of regular ham because I like it more and find that it does a better job wrapping the chicken. I also like using thighs more than chicken breast because they're more flavorful, don't dry out as easily, and are much cheaper—so you actually get more for your money. Any of the recipes in this book that call for chicken breast could easily be substituted with thighs if you discover you love them as much as I do. **SERVES 4**

PREP TIME: 15 minutes
COOK TIME: 45 minutes

3 shallots

2 garlic cloves

8 boneless skinless chicken thighs

Freshly ground black pepper

8 slices prosciutto

2 tablespoons extra-virgin olive oil

PALEO PAIR: Serve with Ginger-Garlic Brussels Sprout Stir-Fry (page 187).

1. Preheat the oven to 300°F.

2. In a food processor or blender, blend the shallots and garlic until they form a paste.

3. On a platter, lay the chicken thighs out flat, and season each piece with pepper. Spoon the garlic and shallot paste evenly onto each thigh, and then roll them as tightly as possible.

4. Wrap each roll with a slice of prosciutto.

5. In a large skillet over medium-high heat, heat the olive oil. Quickly sear the chicken thighs until brown, 2 to 3 minutes on each side.

6. Transfer to a baking dish, and bake for about 40 minutes, or until the chicken is cooked all the way through.

7. Serve immediately.

VARIATION 1 **ARTICHOKE CHICKEN WRAPPED IN PROSCIUTTO:** Add a can of artichoke hearts to the chicken in the baking dish before you put it in the oven.

VARIATION 2 **BBQ BACON-WRAPPED CHICKEN WITH APPLESAUCE:** Brush 8 chicken thighs with 1 cup BBQ Sauce (page 131) before wrapping each with a slice or two of bacon. Cover with about 12 ounces unsweetened applesauce (I like Trader Joe's organic unsweetened applesauce—it comes in a 24-ounce jar). Bake as directed in step 6 of the original recipe. You can also make this recipe in a slow cooker, layering the bacon-wrapped chicken on the bottom and topping with the BBQ Sauce and applesauce. Cook for 8 hours on low, or 3 to 4 hours on high if you're pressed for time.

BUFFALO CHICKEN LEGS

My husband and I are big Buffalo chicken fans. For years, a really fun family night has involved meeting up with my brother for an evening of frying up diced chicken breasts and tossing them with wing sauce to serve alongside homemade French fries. Rob and I love this simple sauce—just two ingredients!—and we've switched from chicken breast to the flavorful, cheap, and pretty underrated chicken leg. **SERVES 2**

PREP TIME: 5 minutes
COOK TIME: 25 minutes

1 tablespoon ghee

5 chicken legs (about 1 pound)

Salt

Freshly ground black pepper

½ cup Frank's Red Hot

½ cup grass-fed butter

1. Preheat the oven to 400°F.

2. In a large ovenproof skillet over medium-high heat, heat the ghee. Season the chicken legs with salt and pepper, and then brown them in the skillet for 5 to 7 minutes on each side.

3. In a small saucepan, heat the hot sauce over low heat. Slowly add in the butter, and stir until it is fully incorporated.

4. Ladle about 1 tablespoon of the Buffalo sauce onto each chicken leg, and transfer the skillet to the oven. Bake for 10 minutes, turning the chicken over halfway through the cooking time.

5. Serve hot with extra Buffalo sauce on the side.

VARIATION 1 **ASIAN CHICKEN LEGS:** Mix together 4 tablespoons honey, 2 minced garlic cloves, ⅓ cup sesame oil, and ⅓ cup coconut aminos and pour over the chicken before baking. Garnish with 2 tablespoons sliced scallions.

VARIATION 2 **BBQ CHICKEN LEGS:** Use homemade BBQ Sauce (page 131) instead of Buffalo sauce if you like a tangier taste.

PALEO PAIR: Serve with Kale Salad with Onion and Avocado (page 128).

PANTRY BASIC: HOMEMADE MAYO

Mayo is one of those things that seems like it's not Paleo, and it's not really, because it's full of soy or canola oil—unless you make it yourself. It might sound impressive, but it's just five ingredients and maybe ten minutes of your time. Mix it with your favorite spices and Paleo sauces to create aiolis, which are delicious spooned over vegetables or for dipping sweet potato fries. The possibilities are endless. **MAKES 1¼ CUPS**

PREP TIME: 10 minutes
COOK TIME: None

1 egg, at room temperature

2 tablespoons freshly squeezed lemon juice, at room temperature

½ teaspoon salt

1 teaspoon dried mustard

1¼ cups light olive oil, divided

1. In a food processor or blender, quickly blitz the egg, lemon juice, salt, mustard, and ¼ cup of olive oil for just a few seconds.

2. Turn the food processor back on, and keep it running while you slowly drizzle in the remaining 1 cup of olive oil. When you have about ⅛ cup left, pour it all in quickly. Transfer to a mason jar or other container with a tightly fitting lid.

3. Store refrigerated until the expiration date of the eggs you use to make it—make a note on the mayo container if it helps you remember.

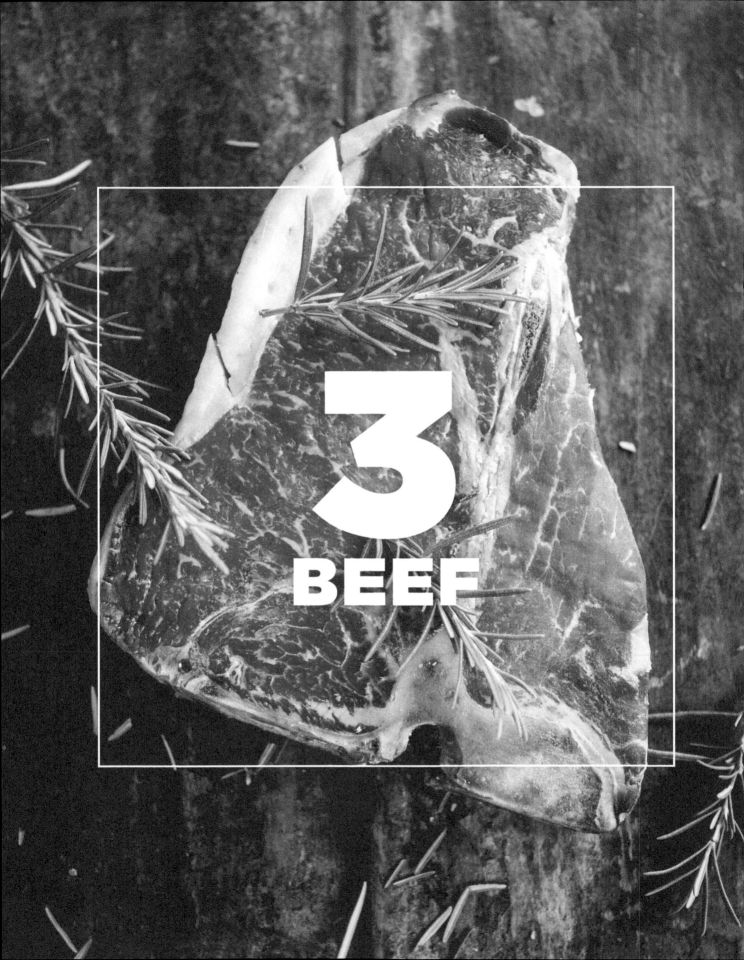

3
BEEF

From steaks to burgers to stir-fries, the preparation possibilities and flavor combinations of beef are endless. Buying a pound of grass-fed ground beef every week is great, because I don't ever have to plan what I'm going to do with it— it can end up in a one-pot veggie-and-beef stir-fry, taco salad, meatballs, or burger bowls.

Some people give up on Paleo because they can't find or afford grass-fed beef (or free-range chicken or eggs, or even organic veggies), but my advice is to do your best with what you can find or afford. Making a stir-fry with conventionally raised and fed beef is a lot better than throwing together some macaroni and cheese, so don't get discouraged! This chapter will give you lots of ideas for not just ground beef, but also tenderloin, flank steaks, and a classic pot roast that I love to make for a crowd on a weekend night or prep ahead for a weeknight dinner.

MEATBALLS

I think meatballs were the first dish to give me what I now refer to as "flour rage," which is when you go Paleo and suddenly realize how much gluten, sugar, and dairy are in foods that really don't need them. Milk in scrambled eggs; sugar in every sauce you'll ever encounter; breadcrumbs in meatballs—sure, it gives them a great texture, but you can make a delicious meatball without any grains or gluten. Here's how! **SERVES 4**

PREP TIME: 10 minutes
COOK TIME: 20 minutes

1 pound ground beef

½ onion, chopped

½ cup chopped fresh parsley, plus 1 tablespoon for garnish

3 garlic cloves, finely chopped

1 egg, beaten

½ teaspoon dried basil

½ teaspoon dried oregano

½ teaspoon salt

½ teaspoon freshly ground black pepper

1 to 2 tablespoons extra-virgin olive oil

1. In a large bowl, stir together the beef, onion, ½ cup of parsley, garlic, egg, basil, oregano, salt, and pepper until thoroughly combined. Using your hands, pinch off palm-size pieces of the mixture and roll into meatballs. You'll end up with 8 to 10 meatballs.

2. In a large frying pan over medium heat, heat the olive oil. Carefully add the meatballs to the pan, and brown on all surfaces, about 5 minutes per side.

3. Remove from the heat, garnish with the remaining 1 tablespoon of parsley, and serve.

VARIATION 1 **MEATBALLS IN TOMATO SAUCE:** After browning the meatballs, add a can of tomato sauce, or make your own from a can of diced tomatoes, ¼ teaspoon garlic powder, salt, and pepper. Simmer for about 10 minutes, and serve.

VARIATION 2 **SLOW COOKER MEATBALLS:** Make these in the morning, and have them ready at the end of the day. Simply layer the uncooked meatballs across the bottom of the slow cooker and cover with tomato sauce. Cook on low for 8 hours.

PALEO PAIR: Serve these meatballs on top of zucchini noodles with tomato sauce. If you don't feel like zucchini, I actually love meatballs on top of Bacon Brussels Sprouts (page 178).

BURGER BOWLS

My family and I make burger bowls whenever we have a big crowd over, especially in the summer. It doesn't take a ton of work, and everyone can customize their own burger. We tend to go all out on toppings, which include (but are never limited to) jalapeños, roasted red peppers, avocado, sautéed mushrooms, tomatoes, onion, and lots of lettuce, which is more of a base than a topping, but important nonetheless. **SERVES 4**

PREP TIME: 10 minutes
COOK TIME: 15 minutes

1 pound ground beef

½ onion, finely chopped, plus ½ onion, sliced, for topping

2 tablespoons homemade Ketchup (page 215)

Salt

Freshly ground black pepper

1 teaspoon extra-virgin olive oil

4 cups field greens or other lettuce

Homemade Mayo (page 47), for topping

Mustard, for topping

Pickles, for topping

Tomatoes, sliced, for topping

1. In a large bowl, stir together the beef, finely chopped onion, and Ketchup until thoroughly combined. Season with salt and pepper. Divide the mixture four ways and form into patties with your hands.

2. Grease a large skillet or grill pan with the olive oil, and cook the burgers over medium heat for 5 to 7 minutes on each side for medium (2 minutes less for rare and 2 minutes more for medium-well).

3. Divide the field greens evenly among 4 serving bowls, and place 1 burger on top of each pile of greens. Top each burger with some onion slices, Homemade Mayo or Ketchup, mustard, pickles, sliced tomatoes, or any other toppings you prefer, and serve.

VARIATION 1 **BACON-MUSHROOM BURGER BOWLS:** Top each burger bowl with ¼ cup Perfect Sautéed Mushrooms (page 207) and 1 or 2 tablespoons cooked and chopped bacon.

VARIATION 2 **BÁNH MÌ BURGER BOWLS:** Substitute the beef with ground pork (the cook time should be about the same), and skip the ketchup. Top with shredded carrots, cucumber, radishes, jalapeños, a drizzle of sesame oil, and some kimchi.

PALEO PAIR: Serve with Chili-Lime Sweet Potato Fries (page 218).

TACO SALAD

If you come over to our house and I wasn't expecting you, I'll probably try to feed you this taco salad. It's one of my favorite easy recipes, and I never get sick of it (probably because it's topped with avocado, salsa, and lime—three of my favorite things). I almost always have the ingredients on hand because, in my opinion, it's just an amalgamation of Paleo staples. Onion, garlic, ground beef—the only thing you may not have in your kitchen right now is taco seasoning, but that's easy enough to obtain (and if you had to go without it, this recipe would still be delicious). **SERVES 4**

PREP TIME: 5 minutes
COOK TIME: 15 minutes

1 to 2 tablespoons extra-virgin olive oil

½ onion, diced

1 or 2 garlic cloves, minced

1 pound ground beef

¼ cup cherry tomatoes (optional)

1 tablespoon taco seasoning

Freshly ground black pepper

2 to 3 cups chopped romaine lettuce, or the salad mix of your choice

4 to 6 tablespoons your favorite Paleo salsa, for garnish

1 avocado, diced or simply quartered, for garnish

1 lime, cut into wedges, for garnish

1. In a large pan over medium heat, heat the olive oil. Sauté the onion until slightly translucent, about 5 minutes. Add the garlic, and cook for another minute.

2. Add the ground beef. Stir it around until it begins to brown, and cook all the way through, 5 to 7 minutes. If there's a lot of liquid, carefully drain it off and return the pan to the heat.

3. Add the cherry tomatoes (if using), and cook for another 2 to 3 minutes, or until they start to get wilty and some of them begin to burst. Stir in the taco seasoning, season with pepper, and remove the pan from the heat.

4. Divide the lettuce evenly among 4 bowls, and top each lettuce pile with the ground beef mixture. Garnish each salad with the salsa, avocado, and lime, and serve.

VARIATION 1 **CHICKEN TACO SALAD:** If you're temporarily tired of beef, recreate this recipe with ground chicken instead (the cook time should be about the same).

VARIATION 2 **SHRIMP TACO SALAD:** Looking for a seafood meal? Use a pound of peeled and deveined shrimp with the tails removed instead of beef and cook until pink (the cook time will be a few minutes shorter).

PREP TIP: Cook the ground beef and chop the veggies on Sunday evening so you're ready for a Monday or Tuesday taco salad dinner.

HAMBURGER AND RICE-STYLE GROUND BEEF

When I was younger, my mom would make hamburger and rice all the time—it was one of my dad's favorite meals, and my brother and I grew to love it as well. Some people who follow the Paleo diet swear by white rice as an acceptable side dish (usually if you're working out enough to justify the carbs), and I occasionally agree; however, the beef and veggies here are satisfying enough on their own, so I serve this recipe as is, or maybe with an extra side of vegetables. **SERVES 4**

PREP TIME: 10 minutes
COOK TIME: 15 minutes

30 **DF** **NF**

1 to 2 tablespoons extra-virgin olive oil

4 roasted red peppers, diced

3 carrots, diced

3 garlic cloves, minced

1 green bell pepper, diced

1 onion, diced

1½ pounds ground beef

4 tablespoons tomato paste

¼ teaspoon red pepper flakes

Salt

Freshly ground black pepper

1 to 2 tablespoons sliced scallion, for garnish

1. In a large skillet over medium heat, heat the olive oil. Sauté the red peppers, carrots, garlic, bell pepper, and onion for 5 to 7 minutes.

2. When everything is slightly browned, raise the heat to medium-high and add the ground beef. Cook for 5 to 7 more minutes, or until browned. Add the tomato paste and red pepper flakes, season with salt and pepper, and stir until everything is incorporated.

3. Keep warm over low heat until ready to serve. Scoop into bowls, and sprinkle with the scallions.

VARIATION 1 **ONE-POT GROUND BEEF AND ASPARAGUS:** Snap off and discard the tough ends of 1 bunch asparagus, chop, and sauté with the rest of the veggies. Continue with the rest of the recipe as written from step 2.

VARIATION 2 **TURKEY HAMBURGER:** Replace the beef with ground turkey for a lighter meal, cooking until no pink remains (the cook time should be about the same).

PALEO PAIR: Serve on top of Shaved Brussels Sprout Salad with Apple Cider Vinaigrette (page 179).

SHEPHERD'S PIE

There are so many great things you can do with cauliflower (which is why we have an entire chapter devoted to it), but one of my favorites is to mash it up with some garlic and butter and use it in place of potatoes. This Paleo Shepherd's Pie does just that, and it's a quick, easy, and welcome change from the everyday ground beef stir-fry that I probably make once a week when I haven't planned our meals well enough. It also looks like it's taken a lot more effort to make than it actually does! **SERVES 4**

PREP TIME: 10 minutes
COOK TIME: 45 minutes

NF

FOR THE FILLING

1 tablespoon extra-virgin olive oil

½ onion, grated

1 or 2 garlic cloves, grated

2 celery stalks, diced

2 or 3 large carrots, diced

1 pound ground beef

Salt

Freshly ground black pepper

2 tablespoons tomato paste

1 teaspoon dried mustard

1 teaspoon dried thyme

½ fresh rosemary sprig, chopped

1 cup chicken broth

1 cup green peas (thawed if frozen)

FOR THE TOPPING

1 large head cauliflower, cut into florets

2 tablespoons grass-fed butter

1 teaspoon garlic powder

Salt

Freshly ground black pepper

1 to 2 tablespoons coconut milk (optional)

TO MAKE THE FILLING

1. In a large pan over medium heat, heat the olive oil. Sauté the onion and garlic until the onion is slightly translucent, about 5 minutes. Add the celery and carrots, and cook for 5 more minutes.

2. Add the ground beef, and season with salt and pepper. Allow to brown, about 5 minutes, and then add the tomato paste, mustard, thyme, and rosemary. Cook for about 10 more minutes, or until any liquid in the pan begins to evaporate.

3. Add the chicken broth, cook for 5 to 7 minutes to reduce it a bit, and then add the peas. Give it a quick stir, and transfer the mixture into one baking dish or individual ramekins.

TO MAKE THE TOPPING

1. While the filling is cooking, fill a large saucepan with water and bring it to a boil. Add the cauliflower to the boiling water, and cook until it is fork-tender, about 10 minutes. Drain the cauliflower and return to the pan.

2. Add the butter and garlic powder, and season with salt and pepper. Use a mixer or immersion blender to mash the cauliflower until it is mostly smooth. If it is too thick, add some coconut milk.

TO ASSEMBLE THE SHEPHERD'S PIE

1. Spread the mashed cauliflower evenly over the beef, and brush the top with the additional ½ tablespoon of melted butter. Place under the broiler for about 5 minutes, or until the mashed cauliflower becomes golden-brown.

2. Serve garnished with the scallions.

FOR ASSEMBLING THE SHEPHERD'S PIE

½ tablespoon melted butter, for brushing

2 tablespoons sliced scallions, for garnish

VARIATION 1 **SHEPHERD'S PIE–STUFFED SWEET POTATOES:** Skip the cauliflower topping and make the filling according to the original recipe. Pierce 4 sweet potatoes with a fork 5 or 6 times each, and place them on a baking sheet. Drizzle with olive oil and season with salt and pepper before baking at 400°F until fork-tender, 45 minutes to 1 hour. Halve the sweet potatoes lengthwise, and scoop out some of the sweet potato flesh to form hollow boats. Fill the hollows with shepherd's pie filling, and serve the scooped-out sweet potato flesh on the side or on top.

VARIATION 2 **LAMB SHEPHERD'S PIE:** Make a more traditional, and slightly gamier-tasting, version of this recipe by swapping out the ground beef for ground lamb (the cook time should be about the same).

PALEO PAIR: Serve with a large helping of Perfect Sautéed Mushrooms (page 207).

BEEF TENDERLOIN

Beef tenderloin is one of my favorite meals—my mom and I make it for almost every party we ever host. It's an impressive dish to look at, but not too fussy to make. All you need to do is season the meat and cook it in the oven. Sliced thinly and presented on a big platter topped with mushrooms or fresh rosemary, it's always greeted with enthusiasm. **SERVES 4 TO 6**

PREP TIME: 10 minutes
COOK TIME: 35 minutes
TOTAL TIME: 1 hour

1 (3-pound) beef tenderloin

3 tablespoons extra-virgin olive oil

3 garlic cloves, minced

Salt

Freshly ground black pepper

2 cups arugula, for serving

1. Preheat the oven to 500°F.

2. Remove the beef from the refrigerator about half an hour before you want to cook it, to bring it to room temperature. Place it in a roasting pan. In a small bowl, stir the olive oil and garlic into a paste. Season with salt and pepper. Coat the tenderloin with the garlic paste, rubbing it in well with your hands. Roast for 15 minutes, or until browned.

3. Lower the heat to 375°F, and cook for another 20 minutes, or until it reaches your desired level of doneness. Use a meat thermometer to be sure (internal temperature of 145°F for medium-rare and 160°F for medium).

4. Rest the beef for 10 to 15 minutes before slicing thinly and serving on a bed of arugula.

VARIATION 1 **BEEF TENDERLOIN WITH MUSHROOMS:** Top the tenderloin with Perfect Sautéed Mushrooms (page 207) before serving.

VARIATION 2 **HERBY MUSTARD TENDERLOIN:** Finely grate ¼ onion and mix it with 2 tablespoons dried mustard and ¼ cup chopped fresh tarragon or rosemary. Rub the tenderloin with the spread, and cook according to the original recipe.

PALEO PAIR: Serve with Broccoli-Arugula Salad with Bacon (page 138).

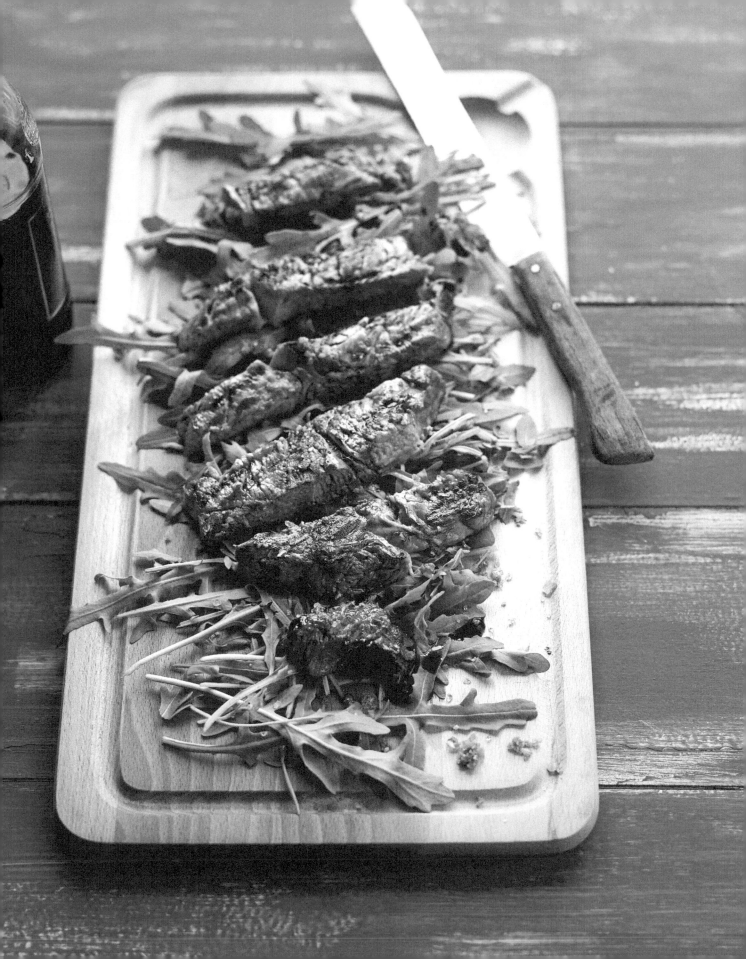

CLASSIC POT ROAST

A pot roast is a great classic weeknight dinner that you really can't go wrong with, whether it's just a couple of you for dinner or you have guests over. This one-pot dinner is tasty and comforting, and just about any vegetable goes well with it. It makes for great leftovers as well, since the flavor of the pork can be paired with any number of side dishes or vegetables. I like to make a big batch, serve it for dinner on Sunday night, and then portion the rest as lunches for the week. **SERVES 4 TO 6**

PREP TIME: 10 minutes
COOK TIME: 3 hours

1 (3- to 4-pound) boneless chuck roast

Salt

Freshly ground black pepper

2 tablespoons extra-virgin olive oil

1 onion, sliced

2 garlic cloves, minced

2 celery stalks, diced

½ cup red wine (optional; omit if strict Paleo)

1 cup beef broth

2 or 3 dried bay leaves

2 or 3 fresh thyme sprigs

4 carrots, chopped

1 cup green peas (thawed if frozen)

PREP TIP: Pressed for time? After searing the meat in step 2, just cook everything in the oven at once for 2½ hours.

1. Preheat the oven to 350°F.

2. Season the roast with salt and pepper. In an ovenproof pot (such as a Dutch oven) over high heat, heat the olive oil. Sear the meat for 3 to 5 minutes per side. Remove the roast from the pot, and set aside.

3. Add the onion, garlic, and celery to the pot, and sauté until the onion is slightly translucent, about 5 minutes. Pour in the wine (if using), and stir it around to deglaze the pot, scraping up any browned bits from the bottom.

4. Place the roast on top of the vegetables, and add the beef broth, bay leaves, and thyme. Put the pot into the oven, and cook for 1½ hours.

5. Add the carrots, and cook for an additional hour. Make sure the liquid hasn't all evaporated; if it has, add a bit more.

6. Remove the pot from the oven, and add the peas. Cover the pot, and allow the peas to cook for 10 minutes while the meat rests in the dish.

7. Serve immediately.

VARIATION 1 **SWEET POTATO POT ROAST:** Add 2 medium sweet potatoes, peeled and cubed, to the pot when you add the carrots in step 5.

VARIATION 2 **SLOW COOKER ROAST:** Sear the roast as instructed in step 2, and then place all the ingredients (except for the peas) in the slow cooker. Cook for 8 hours on low, and add the peas 10 minutes before serving.

ROPA VIEJA

If you haven't been to Miami, you should go, and eat Cuban food every day—it's wonderful. I had ropa vieja for the first time at a Cuban restaurant in Miami, and I really liked it. The dish got its name because *ropa vieja* means "old clothes" in Spanish, and the strips of beef, peppers, and onions apparently resemble colorful shredded rags. It's not the most appetizing image, but I promise this recipe is delicious. **SERVES 4**

PREP TIME: 10 minutes
COOK TIME: 1 hour, 15 minutes

DF NF

1 to 2 tablespoons extra-virgin olive oil

2 to 3 pounds flank steak

1 red onion, sliced

4 garlic cloves, minced

2 red bell peppers, cut into strips

2 green bell peppers, cut into strips

1 teaspoon dried oregano

1 teaspoon ground cumin

¼ cup sherry vinegar

3 cups beef broth

1 tablespoon tomato paste

2 dried bay leaves

Salt

Freshly ground black pepper

½ cup chopped fresh cilantro, for garnish

PREP TIP: Cook everything ahead of time, and leave the hour of simmering for when you're almost ready to serve.

1. In a large Dutch oven or pot over medium-high heat, heat the olive oil. Brown the beef (you may need to cut it in half and work in batches), about 3 minutes per side. Set aside.

2. Reduce the heat to medium, and add the onion, garlic, and red and green bell peppers to the pot. Stirring frequently, cook for 5 to 7 minutes, until tender. Add the oregano and cumin, and cook for 1 minute more.

3. Add the sherry vinegar, and deglaze the pan, stirring up any browned bits from the bottom. Cook for a couple of minutes, until most of the liquid has evaporated. Add the broth and tomato paste, and stir well to combine. Throw in the bay leaves, and return the beef to the pot. Season with salt and pepper. Bring the whole thing to a simmer, reduce the heat to low, and cook for another hour.

4. Transfer the meat to a platter, and shred it. Return the meat to the stew, stir, and serve garnished with the cilantro.

VARIATION 1 **CHICKEN ROPA VIEJA WITH OLIVES:** Make this recipe with chicken instead of beef. Shred 2 to 3 pounds cooked boneless skinless chicken breast. Continue with the recipe as written from step 2, but stir ¼ cup sliced green olives into the stew before serving.

VARIATION 2 **SLOW COOKER ROPA VIEJA:** In a large skillet over high heat, brown the beef. Transfer to a slow cooker, along with the remaining ingredients, and cook on low for 8 to 10 hours. Transfer the beef to a platter, and allow it to cool slightly. Shred the beef, return it to the slow cooker, stir, and serve.

VACA FRITA

Over the years I've discovered that my favorite foods are generally those that do well with a generous squeeze of fresh lime juice—pad thai, tacos, and a lot of Latin dishes like this one. *Vaca frita* translated into English means "fried cow," and it's exactly what it sounds like—delicious beef prepared on the stove and then fried until crispy. **SERVES 4**

PREP TIME: 10 minutes
COOK TIME: 1 hour
TOTAL TIME: 1 hour, 40 minutes

NF

2 pounds flank steak

1 dried bay leaf

2 onions, 1 quartered and the other sliced

2 tablespoons grass-fed butter

2 garlic cloves, smashed

¼ cup freshly squeezed lime juice, plus 1 lime, quartered, for garnish

3 to 4 tablespoons extra-virgin olive oil, divided

Salt

Freshly ground black pepper

PALEO PAIR: Vaca frita is traditionally served with white rice and some beans, so to complete the meal, serve it with a side of Cauliflower Fried Rice (page 116).

1. In a large pot, cover the flank steak (you may need to cut it in half or even quarters), bay leaf, and quartered onion with enough water to cover the meat by an inch. Bring to a boil, and then simmer over low heat for 20 minutes.

2. While the beef is cooking, in a medium skillet over medium-low heat, heat the butter. Gently cook the sliced onion until it is very soft and dark brown, about 20 minutes.

3. When the beef finishes cooking, transfer it to a platter and allow it to cool before using your hands to shred it into very thin pieces.

4. Transfer the shredded beef to a large bowl, and add the garlic and lime juice. Mix well, and then allow it to marinate for 30 minutes on the counter.

5. In a large skillet over high heat, heat 1 tablespoon of olive oil. Working in batches, fry the shredded beef in a single layer until very browned and crispy, 4 to 7 minutes per batch. Season with salt and pepper, and remove from the heat. Repeat with the rest of the beef, adding more oil as necessary.

6. Serve each plate of vaca frita topped with some of the sautéed onions and a wedge of fresh lime.

VARIATION 1 **VACA FRITA DE POLLO:** Make this recipe with chicken instead of beef, and cook it the same way (in a pot with a dried bay leaf, onion, and water), but for about 40 minutes instead of 20. Continue with the recipe as written from step 2.

VARIATION 2 **VACA FRITA WITH FRIED ONIONS:** If you don't want to caramelize the onions, throw them into the bowl with the beef (in step 4), and then fry everything together.

STEAK MARSALA

At first I thought it would be hard to find something Paleo to eat at an Italian restaurant, but it's really not too bad if you do a little digging past the pasta and lasagna. I love to order steak Marsala if it's on the menu, and I get a side of vegetables instead of pasta. It's always delicious, but I know the sauce is probably full of flour, so I decided to make a Paleo version of my own. It's really easy—you just make the sauce and serve it with your favorite steak. **SERVES 4**

PREP TIME: 10 minutes
COOK TIME: 35 minutes
TOTAL TIME: 55 minutes

`DF` `NF`

FOR THE SAUCE
3 tablespoons extra-virgin olive oil
½ onion, sliced
10 ounces mushrooms
2 garlic cloves, minced
½ cup Marsala wine
1½ cups beef broth
Salt
Freshly ground black pepper

FOR THE STEAKS
4 large steaks (rib eyes or sirloin)
4 tablespoons grass-fed butter

PALEO PAIR: Serve with Whole Roasted Cauliflower (page 113).

TO MAKE THE SAUCE

1. In a medium saucepan over medium heat, heat the olive oil. Sauté the onion until slightly translucent, about 5 minutes. Add the mushrooms and garlic, and cook for another 5 minutes.

2. Add the Marsala wine, and deglaze the pan, scraping up any browned bits from the bottom, and add the beef broth. Season with salt and pepper, and cook down until the sauce begins to thicken, 8 to 10 minutes. Reduce the heat to low, and simmer until ready to serve.

TO COOK THE STEAKS

1. Preheat the oven to 400°F.

2. In a large ovenproof skillet over high heat, sear the steaks for 2 to 3 minutes per side, until browned. Transfer to the oven, and cook for 6 to 10 minutes, depending on how rare you want them. Remove from the oven, and place 1 tablespoon of butter on each steak.

3. Let rest for 10 minutes before slicing. Top with the Marsala sauce, and serve.

VARIATION 1 **CHICKEN MARSALA:** Brown the chicken in a large pan for 4 to 5 minutes on each side, and then pour the Marsala sauce over it. Simmer on low in the sauce until cooked through, about 10 to 15 more minutes.

VARIATION 2 **LAMB CHOP MARSALA:** Season 4 lamb chops with salt and pepper, and then sear them in a very hot cast iron pan for 3 to 5 minutes per side (flipping once). Then cook for an additional 5 minutes, or until cooked to your liking (medium or medium-rare is best). Serve with the Marsala sauce.

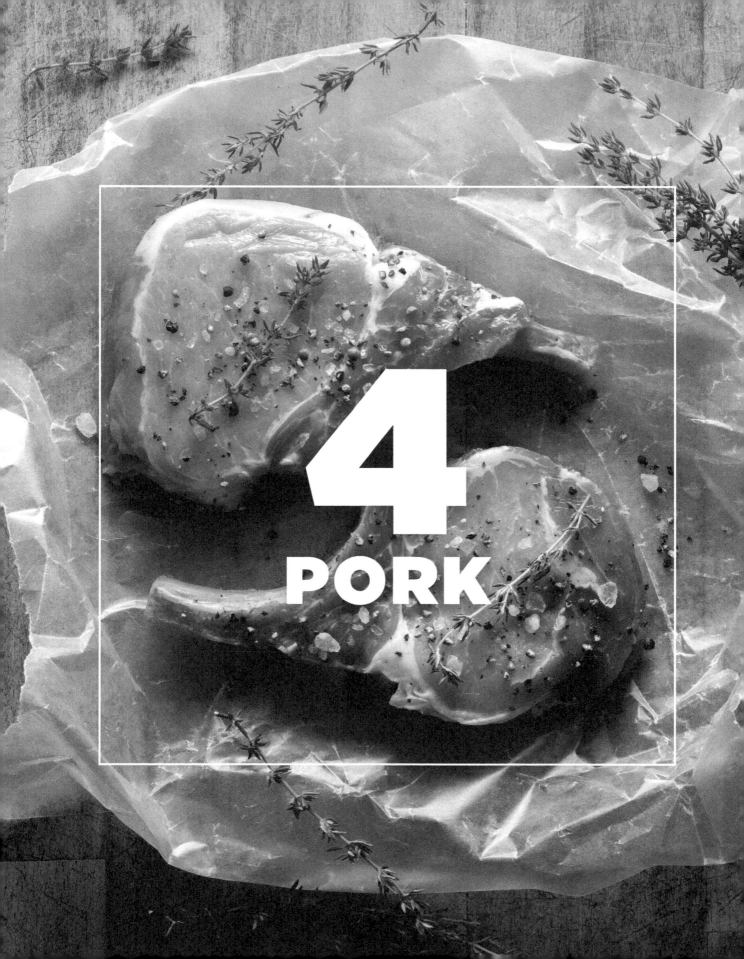

4
PORK

I don't usually cook pork as a main dish, but I have been known to use a little too much bacon in my cooking. In this chapter I've included one of my favorite appetizer recipes of all time—Sausage-Stuffed Dates Wrapped in Bacon (page 64)—as well as some pretty solid lunch options like Bánh Mì Tacos (page 68) and Sesame Pork Salad (page 66). Pork lends itself so well to Asian flavors.

Pork is great for plan-ahead meals that make dinner super quick, like Pulled Pork BBQ (page 74), which I love to make in the slow cooker. A lot of my pork recipes call for low, slow heat; I've found that preparing it that way keeps it from drying out, and I like coming home from a long day to a dinner that's already mostly done. If you don't have a slow cooker, don't fret—your oven is more than sufficient; just ask my brother and his Baby Back Ribs recipe (page 70).

SAUSAGE-STUFFED DATES WRAPPED IN BACON

I've been wrapping dates in bacon since 2012, when I first encountered the dish at Más Tapas, my favorite restaurant in Charlottesville, Virginia. Those were stuffed with goat cheese, which is delicious, but if you don't tolerate dairy, you can just make them without it. We started experimenting with different fillings and finally landed on this one: sausage. They can be a little time-consuming to make, but they are totally worth it. **SERVES 8 TO 10**

PREP TIME: 15 minutes
COOK TIME: 30 minutes

16 to 20 dates, pitted

1 pound spicy ground pork sausage

8 to 10 slices bacon, halved

1. Preheat the oven to 400°F.

2. Carefully slice each date down the middle (but not all the way through—just enough so that you can stuff it with sausage).

3. Roll out tablespoon-size ovals of sausage in your hand. Stuff each date with a sausage oval. Wrap each stuffed date with half a strip of bacon, and place it on a baking sheet.

4. Bake the dates for 20 to 30 minutes, or until the bacon is crispy and the sausage is cooked through, and serve.

VARIATION 1 **ALMOND-STUFFED BACON DATES:** Instead of sausage, stuff each date with an almond. Wrap with bacon, and bake as instructed.

VARIATION 2 **BACON-WRAPPED DATES WITH APPLE CIDER VINAIGRETTE:** In a medium bowl, stir to combine 1 tablespoon minced shallot with 1 to 2 tablespoons honey, ¼ cup apple cider vinegar, and ½ cup olive oil. Drizzle over the bacon-wrapped dates after cooking, and serve. Keep any leftover dressing in the fridge to use on salads.

PALEO PAIR: Serve these as appetizers along with Bacon Brussels Sprouts (page 178) and Bacon-Wrapped Shrimp (page 92) at your next party.

CANDIED BACON SALAD

Remember when bacon was A Thing? It was everywhere. Bacon chocolate, bacon cupcakes . . . I love bacon as much as the next Paleo person, but I'm glad to see that the hype has died down a bit. That doesn't mean I'm not going to freak out about this candied bacon, though. It's really more of a garnish than anything else, which is why I came up with this sweet and tangy salad that is the perfect vehicle for it. **SERVES 4**

PREP TIME: 5 minutes
COOK TIME: 20 minutes

10 to 12 ounces thick-cut bacon, halved or quartered

½ cup maple syrup

3 to 4 cups field greens (or your favorite salad mix)

½ cup pecans

¼ cup Apple Cider Vinaigrette (page 179)

1. Preheat the oven to 400°F.

2. On a baking sheet, lay out the bacon in a single layer, and brush with the maple syrup. Bake for 15 to 20 minutes, or until the bacon is as crispy as you like it. Chop or crumble the bacon into bite-size pieces.

3. In a large serving bowl, toss the greens with the pecans and Apple Cider Vinaigrette. Top with the candied bacon, and serve.

VARIATION 1 **SPICY CANDIED BACON:** Sprinkle the bacon with ¼ teaspoon ground cayenne pepper before baking.

VARIATION 2 **HONEY CANDIED BACON:** Swap the maple syrup for honey—just drizzle a little on each piece, and rub it in with your hands.

PALEO PAIR: Serve with Coconut Shrimp (page 97).

SESAME PORK SALAD

This salad is a nice, light way to prepare and enjoy pork—the thin strips cook pretty quickly and then go over fresh, crisp lettuce or cucumber noodles. I love Asian flavors with pork, and I'm always trying to come up with salad ideas that aren't boring, so this one is always welcome in my meal planning rotation. **SERVES 4**

PREP TIME: 10 minutes, plus 20 minutes to marinate
COOK TIME: 10 minutes

2 tablespoons honey

2 tablespoons sesame oil

1 tablespoon coconut aminos

½ tablespoon chili oil

½ tablespoon fish sauce

½ onion, diced

2 garlic cloves, minced

¼ to ½ teaspoon freshly ground black pepper

1 pound pork cutlets, cut into strips

2 to 3 cups chopped romaine (or your favorite salad lettuce)

1 or 2 tablespoons sesame seeds, for garnish

1. In a large bowl, stir to combine the honey, sesame oil, coconut aminos, chili oil, fish sauce, onion, garlic, and pepper. Add the pork, and marinate for at least 20 minutes.

2. Heat a cast iron pan or skillet over high heat. Add the pork, and cook until seared on all sides, about 10 minutes.

3. Put the chopped lettuce in a large serving bowl, and top it with the cooked pork. Garnish with the sesame seeds, and serve.

VARIATION 1 SESAME PORK SALAD WITH CUCUMBER NOODLES: Use a spiralizer to make cucumber noodles, and serve the pork over that instead of lettuce. If you don't have a spiralizer or vegetable peeler, you can julienne a cucumber with a knife.

VARIATION 2 SESAME PORK WITH SHREDDED CABBAGE: For a slightly stronger taste and more of a crunch, serve the pork over shredded cabbage instead of lettuce or cucumber noodles.

PREP TIP: Make an extra serving of marinade, and use it as salad dressing; just make sure it doesn't go near the raw pork. Discard all marinades that have touched raw meat, as potentially dangerous bacteria can easily be transferred.

GROUND PORK STIR-FRY

This is a great weeknight dinner idea using ground pork instead of ground beef, which I usually use. I call it a stir-fry, although it's not very Asian in flavor—I guess you could call it a scramble, although there aren't any eggs in it (unless you try the scramble variation). More than anything, it's just a quick one-pot dish that makes cooking, serving, and clean-up as easy as possible. Like the veggie scramble in the egg chapter, you can add any and all vegetables to this one if you're trying to use up something in your fridge. **SERVES 4**

PREP TIME: 5 minutes
COOK TIME: 20 minutes

1½ tablespoons extra-virgin olive oil or coconut oil

½ onion, diced

1 green bell pepper, cut into strips

10 ounces mushrooms, sliced

1 or 2 small zucchini, diced

3 garlic cloves, minced

1 pound ground pork

Salt

Freshly ground black pepper

¼ teaspoon red pepper flakes

1. In a large frying pan over medium heat, heat the olive oil. Add the onion, and sauté until slightly translucent, about 5 minutes.

2. Add the bell pepper, mushrooms, and zucchini. Allow to cook down for another 5 minutes before adding the garlic.

3. Move all the sautéed vegetables to the outside edges of the pan, and put the ground pork in the middle. Season with salt and pepper, and cook, stirring with a wooden spoon to break up the pieces, until the pork and the garlic begin to brown, about 5 minutes. Stir the vegetables into the center until everything is well mixed. Turn the heat up to medium-high, and cook until some of the pork begins to crisp up, about 5 minutes.

4. Add the red pepper flakes, give it another stir, and serve hot.

VARIATION 1 **STIR-FRY SCRAMBLE:** Right before turning off the heat, crack 2 eggs into the pan and scramble them into the stir-fry for 2 to 3 minutes.

VARIATION 2 **CHICKEN SESAME STIR-FRY:** Use ground chicken instead of pork (cook time should be about the same), and substitute sesame oil for the olive oil. Top with 1 or 2 tablespoons sesame seeds and 2 tablespoons sliced scallions for garnish. This gives the dish a mildly Asian character.

PREP TIP: Use this recipe to get rid of veggies that need to be used before they go bad or get too wilty. Add chopped broccoli, sweet potatoes, spinach, kale, or squash—anything goes!

BÁNH MÌ TACOS

There's a great burger place in Roanoke, Virginia, called Beamer's 25 (named after Virginia Tech football coach Frank Beamer), and I almost always order their Bánh Mì burger, a pork burger topped with pickled veggies and served with a side of ginger. I thought about that burger when I came up with this recipe for Bánh Mì Tacos, which are just a lightened-up version—stir-fried pork bites are seasoned with sesame oil, honey, and red pepper flakes for that delightful spicy-sweet combination, and then we serve them on lettuce leaves topped with quick-pickled veggies. It's a perfect appetizer or light dinner. **SERVES 4**

PREP TIME: 10 minutes, plus 1 hour and 10 minutes to marinate

COOK TIME: 10 minutes

DF **NF**

FOR THE QUICK-PICKLED VEGETABLES

¼ cup white vinegar

1 tablespoon coconut aminos

½ cup carrots, julienned

½ cup cucumber, julienned

3 or 4 radishes, thinly sliced

FOR THE TACOS

2 tablespoons honey

1 tablespoon sesame oil

1 teaspoon white vinegar

¼ teaspoon red pepper flakes

1 pound pork cutlets, cut thinly into bite-size pieces

4 to 6 lettuce leaves, either romaine or butter lettuce

2 or 3 tablespoons chopped fresh cilantro, for garnish

TO MAKE THE QUICK-PICKLED VEGETABLES

In a small bowl, stir to combine the vinegar with the coconut aminos. Add the carrots, cucumber, and radishes. Cover and marinate in the refrigerator for 1 hour.

TO MAKE THE TACOS

1. In a medium bowl, stir to combine the honey, sesame oil, vinegar, and red pepper flakes. Add the pork, and stir. Marinate for 10 minutes.

2. In a large skillet over medium-high heat, sauté the pork in the marinade for 5 to 7 minutes, or until the pork strips are cooked through.

3. Set up your tacos by laying out the lettuce boats and filling them with cooked pork. Top with a generous serving of the quick-pickled vegetables, and garnish with the cilantro.

VARIATION 1 **BÁNH MÌ TACOS WITH SHRIMP:** For a meatless variation, marinate 1 pound peeled and deveined shrimp with the tails removed instead of the pork strips. Cook for 3 to 4 minutes or until pink. Prepare the tacos as written in step 3.

VARIATION 2 **ASIAN PORK BELLY TACOS:** Swap out pork cutlets for pork belly, which has a deliciously rich, fatty taste. Sauté as written in the recipe, and then pour the marinade over it. Continue to cook for 2 to 3 minutes more, and assemble the tacos as written in step 3.

PREP TIP: Make the pickled vegetables ahead of time so you don't end up waiting an hour for them.

CARNITAS

Carnitas is not only super delicious, but also a really versatile main dish that you can repurpose for all kinds of meals, such as tacos or salad bowls, or even enjoy it on its own with a side of vegetables. The cooking time is a bit lengthy, so you need to plan ahead, but if you do that, the active cooking is minimal—almost a set-it-and-forget-it kind of situation, which is always a nice break. If you have any left over, pour the cooking liquid over it to keep it all nice and moist. **SERVES 6**

PREP TIME: 10 minutes
COOK TIME: 2 hours, 30 minutes

2 tablespoons extra-virgin olive oil

1 (2-pound) pork shoulder

Salt

Freshly ground black pepper

3 to 4 cups water

4 garlic cloves, crushed

3 fresh thyme sprigs

2 dried bay leaves

2 teaspoons dried oregano

1. Preheat the oven to 325°F.

2. In a large ovenproof pot or Dutch oven over medium-high heat, heat the olive oil. Season the pork shoulder with salt and pepper, and gently lower it into the pot. Sear for 5 to 7 minutes on each side, or until browned. Add the water, garlic, thyme, bay leaves, and oregano, and transfer the pot to the oven.

3. Cook for 1½ to 2 hours, or until the pork is cooked through and can easily be shredded with a couple of forks. Shred the whole thing, stir it around in the cooking liquid, and serve.

VARIATION 1 **CARNITAS TACO SALAD:** For a different texture, make the Taco Salad (page 52) with the carnitas instead of ground beef.

VARIATION 2 **SLOW COOKER CARNITAS:** Put all the ingredients in a slow cooker, and cook on low for 8 hours.

PREP TIP: Make the carnitas ahead of time, and store in the fridge for up to 5 days or in the freezer for up to 3 months.

BABY BACK RIBS

My brother makes the best ribs I've ever had—it's probably his dry rub, which he was nice enough to share with us here. My husband and I love making ribs on a Sunday when we're going to be home all afternoon and can enjoy the smell of spicy, slow-cooked pork; it's like driving on a summer night past our favorite BBQ place, down the street from our first apartment in Charlotte. **SERVES 4**

PREP TIME: 10 minutes, plus 1 hour to marinate
COOK TIME: 2 hours, 45 minutes

DF **NF**

2 whole slabs pork baby back ribs

¾ cup Dry Rub (page 229)

1 cup white wine or beef broth

2 tablespoons honey

2 tablespoons white vinegar

2 garlic cloves, crushed

1. Line a baking sheet with aluminum foil. Lay the ribs flat on the baking sheet, and sprinkle them with the Dry Rub. Rub it in with your hands. Cover the sheet with more foil, and refrigerate for at least an hour.

2. Preheat the oven to 225°F.

3. In a small saucepan over low heat, mix together the wine or broth, honey, vinegar, and garlic, and warm for about 5 minutes. Open the foil, and pour half of the liquid in under the ribs. Return the pan to the stove, bring to a boil, and then reduce to a simmer.

4. Put the ribs in the oven, and bake for 2½ hours.

5. While the ribs cook, simmer the remaining sauce over low heat so it thickens into a glaze.

6. When the time is up, remove the ribs from the oven, and turn the heat to broil. Drizzle the sauce over the ribs, pop them under the broiler until they're nicely browned, about 5 minutes, and serve.

VARIATION 1 **ASIAN BABY BACK RIBS:** Add 2 tablespoons sesame oil and 1 teaspoon garlic chili paste to the glaze, and garnish the cooked ribs with a sprinkle of sesame seeds and 1 to 2 tablespoons sliced scallions.

VARIATION 2 **BBQ RIBS:** Skip the Dry Rub and the glaze; instead, brush the ribs with homemade BBQ Sauce (page 131) for faster prep. Add 1 tablespoon chopped fresh rosemary for extra flavor (shown, right).

PREP TIP: Keep the rib bones and make bone broth with them (see the Chicken Soup recipe on page 36).

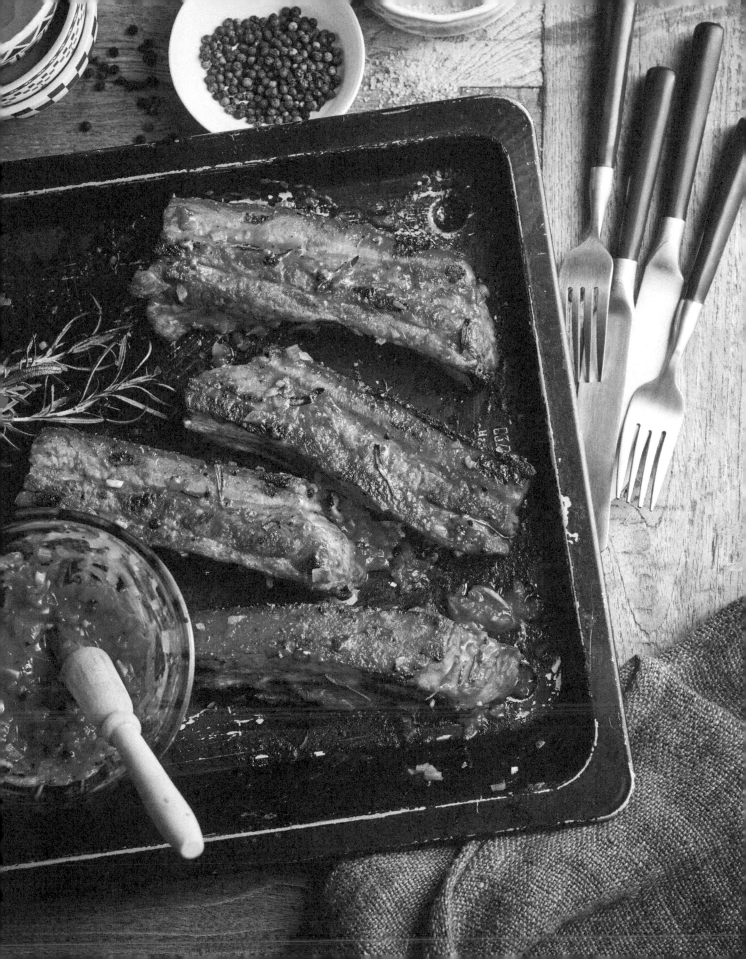

STUFFED PORK CHOPS

My mom and I came up with this recipe one winter when she was visiting me in Charlotte, and we were so pleased with how it turned out that we had to write it down. This stuffed pork chop is especially good in the fall; I love the way the apples, raisins, and cinnamon come together once they've cooked down a little. I add onion to almost everything, so it makes sense that it made its way into this stuffing. **SERVES 4**

PREP TIME: 10 minutes
COOK TIME: 30 minutes

DF **NF**

2 tablespoons extra-virgin olive oil, divided

1 apple, peeled and diced

½ onion, diced

¼ cup raisins (any kind but yellow would be nice)

¼ teaspoon ground cinnamon

¼ teaspoon ground nutmeg

4 thick-cut boneless pork chops

Salt

Freshly ground black pepper

1. Preheat the oven to 375°F.

2. In a large ovenproof skillet over medium heat, heat 1 tablespoon of olive oil. Stir in the apple, onion, and raisins, followed by the cinnamon and nutmeg. Sauté until the onions become slightly translucent, about 5 minutes. Transfer the mixture to a bowl to cool.

3. Slice a pocket into the side of each pork chop, then stuff with the cooled raisin-apple mixture. If you want, you can close the slit with a toothpick, but that's optional; some stuffing might fall out as you cook, but you can just top the pork chops with it later. Season the chops with salt and pepper.

4. Pour the remaining 1 tablespoon of olive oil into the pan, and brown the pork chops for 4 to 5 minutes on each side.

5. Transfer to the oven and bake for 15 to 20 minutes, or until the thickest part of the chop registers 155°F with a meat thermometer, and serve.

VARIATION 1 **GARLIC SPINACH–STUFFED PORK CHOPS:** replace the apple, raisins, cinnamon, and nutmeg with 1 cup well-washed and drained spinach and 2 or 3 minced garlic cloves for a more savory version, and follow the recipe as written.

VARIATION 2 **PAN-FRIED STUFFED PORK CHOPS:** Skip the oven step and finish the pork chops on the stove. Just cook for an additional 10 minutes per side, or until the meat reaches an internal temperature of 155°F.

PALEO PAIR: Serve with Sautéed Squash with Sun-Dried Tomatoes (page 193).

PROSCIUTTO-WRAPPED PORK TENDERLOIN

This is a delicious and kind of fancy dinner recipe that you can make pretty easily for a crowd. It's a pork version of a bacon-wrapped beef tenderloin, and I love the glaze that goes on it. The prosciutto is nice and salty, so you really don't need to add more salt when seasoning the meat. What's great about these kinds of recipes is that they're special without being complicated, so you can make them for either a casual Sunday dinner or a ritzy weekend dinner party. **SERVES 4 TO 6**

PREP TIME: 10 minutes
COOK TIME: 30 minutes
TOTAL TIME: 50 minutes

DF **NF**

4 tablespoons Dijon mustard

3 tablespoons balsamic vinegar

1 tablespoon honey

1 tablespoon fresh thyme leaves

¾ tablespoon fresh rosemary leaves, chopped

1 teaspoon freshly ground black pepper

¼ teaspoon red pepper flakes, or more if desired

3 pounds pork tenderloin

12 slices prosciutto

1. Preheat the oven to 350°F.

2. In a small bowl, whisk to combine the mustard, vinegar, honey, thyme, rosemary, pepper, and red pepper flakes until smooth. Rub half of the mixture all over the tenderloin.

3. In an ovenproof pan over medium-high heat, sear the tenderloin for 2 to 3 minutes per side to caramelize the honey. Remove it from the pan, and allow it to cool slightly. Wrap the tenderloin with the prosciutto, overlapping the slices if necessary.

4. Put the pork back in the pan, and bake for 25 minutes. If the prosciutto isn't crispy by then, run it under the broiler until it is.

5. Let it rest for 5 to 10 minutes before slicing and serving.

VARIATION 1 **SPICY APRICOT SAUCE TENDERLOIN:** In a medium saucepan over medium heat, cook 4 quartered ripe apricots, the juice of 1 orange, ½ teaspoon fresh ginger, ½ teaspoon salt, ½ teaspoon red pepper flakes, 2 tablespoons agave nectar, and some freshly ground black pepper, stirring often, for about 20 minutes. Reduce to low and simmer for another 5 minutes. Allow to cool, and then purée or blend with an immersion blender. Bake the tenderloin at 350°F for 25 minutes, and serve the sauce with the pork.

VARIATION 2 **BACON-WRAPPED PORK TENDERLOIN:** Use bacon instead of prosciutto, and mix together 4 tablespoons Dijon mustard and 2 tablespoons honey for the glaze. Continue with the rest of the recipe as written.

PALEO PAIR: Serve with Shaved Brussels Sprout Salad with Apple Cider Vinaigrette (page 179).

PULLED PORK BBQ

I grew up in Virginia and later moved to North Carolina, so BBQ has been part of my life for as long as I can remember. My family actually moved to Virginia from California, though, so when we first arrived in the South, we were surprised by the difference between "cooking out" and "BBQ." To us, barbecue was what you did when you grilled outside, but we soon learned what BBQ itself was—pulled pork. **SERVES 4 TO 6**

PREP TIME: 10 minutes
COOK TIME: 2 hours, 15 minutes

2 pounds pork butt

1 tablespoon salt

1 tablespoon freshly ground black pepper

2 cups BBQ Sauce (page 131)

1. Preheat the oven to 425°F.

2. On a baking sheet, season the pork with the salt and pepper. Using your hands, spread half of the BBQ sauce all over the meat.

3. Bake for 45 minutes, and then lower the heat to 350°F and bake for another 1½ hours.

4. Remove the pork from the oven, and allow to cool slightly. Transfer the pork to a bowl, and shred with a fork. Add the rest of the BBQ sauce, and serve.

VARIATION 1 **SLOW COOKER BBQ:** This is actually the way I prefer to cook my BBQ: Place the pork in the slow cooker, season with salt and pepper, and then cover with half of sauce as in the original recipe. Cook on low for 8 hours, and then shred it with a fork, right in the slow cooker.

VARIATION 2 **OVEN-ROASTED CHICKEN BBQ:** Grease a baking sheet and place 10 bone-in thighs on it, skin-side down. Bake at 400°F for 25 minutes. Remove from the oven, and brush the exposed side with BBQ sauce. Flip the chicken, brush with more sauce, and bake skin-side up for 7 to 8 minutes more. Remove from the oven again, and brush once more with sauce. Finally, raise the oven temperature to 425°F and bake for 5 to 7 more minutes, or until the skin becomes crunchy.

PALEO PAIR: Serve with Southern-Style Kale Greens (page 124).

PANTRY BASIC: RANCH DRESSING

There are a few things I didn't know I really loved until I gave them up, among them muffins, sandwiches, and ranch dressing. My mom, brother, and I came up with this Paleo ranch when we were making Buffalo chicken one night and lamenting the fact that blue cheese isn't Paleo (important statement: ranch is great, but blue cheese was meant for Buffalo wings). Now I keep a batch of this dressing in my refrigerator to serve on salads or dip veggies into as a snack. **MAKES 1½ CUPS**

PREP TIME: 5 minutes
COOK TIME: None

30 DF NF

1 cup Homemade Mayo
(page 47)

½ cup coconut milk

½ tablespoon dried chives

1 teaspoon dried mustard

½ teaspoon celery seed

½ teaspoon dried dill

½ teaspoon garlic powder

½ teaspoon onion powder

Pinch salt

Pinch freshly ground
black pepper

1. In a mason jar or other container with a tightly fitting lid, shake or mix well to combine the Homemade Mayo, coconut milk, chives, mustard, celery seed, dill, garlic powder, onion powder, salt, and pepper.

2. Store refrigerated until the expiration date of the eggs you used to make the mayo—make a note on the container if it helps you remember.

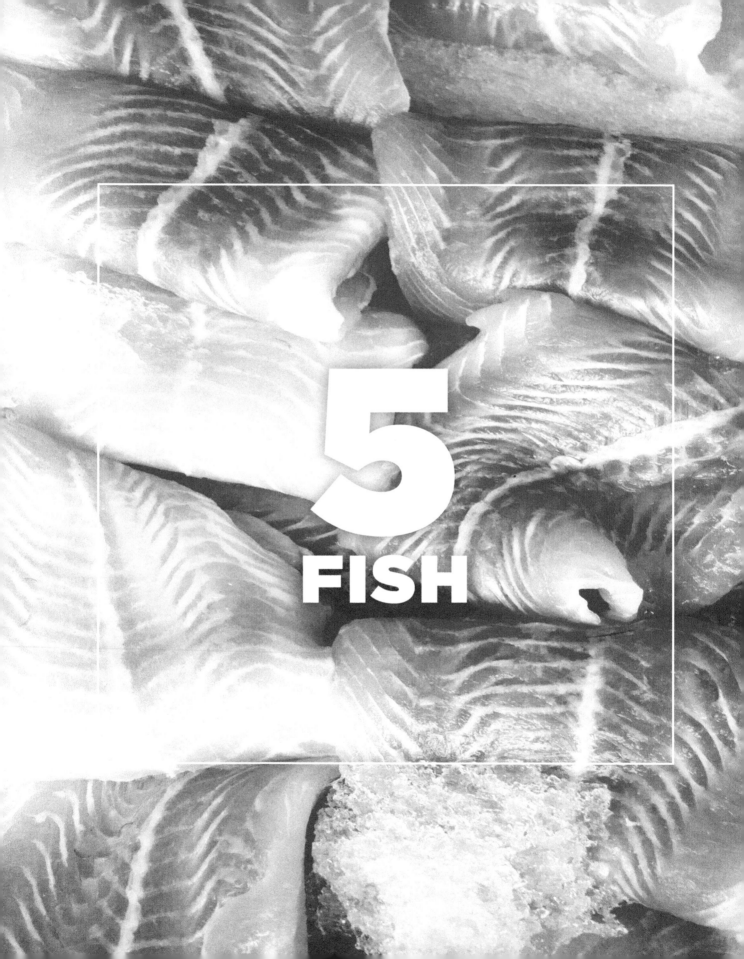

5
FISH

Once every three months or so, my husband and I joke about how rarely we eat fish. We lived in an apartment for years, and something about the smaller space always made us feel like cooking fish on the stove was going to stink up our place for days; so unless we could go outside and grill it, fish was mostly something we ate in restaurants.

But as I've experimented with it more and more over the years, I've come to realize how little cooking time most fish really needs, and what a great option it is. This chapter is full of recipes that cook pretty quickly, and although most of them call for a specific fish, like mahi mahi or sea bass, you can essentially substitute any white, flaky fish.

I hope that if you rarely make fish for yourself or your family at home, this chapter will inspire you to pick up some fillets of halibut or cod the next time you're walking through the grocery store.

LEMON-BUTTER TILAPIA

This is absolutely one of the easiest recipes I've ever made—and it's also one of the most delicious. Sometimes I go a really long time without making fish because I somehow convince myself that it's a hassle, when in reality it's one of the fastest-cooking proteins around. The fish is lightly poached in a simple lemon-butter sauce that makes clean-up easy—perfect for a busy weeknight dinner at home. **SERVES 2**

PREP TIME: 5 minutes
COOK TIME: 15 minutes

2 tablespoons grass-fed butter

1 garlic clove, sliced

2 (6-ounce) tilapia fillets

Salt

Freshly ground black pepper

½ lemon, plus 2 lemon slices for garnish

2 tablespoons chopped fresh parsley, for garnish

1. In a medium sauté pan over low heat, melt the butter. Add the garlic, and simmer for about 5 minutes.

2. Season both sides of the fish with a sprinkle of salt and pepper. Gently place the fillets in the pan, and cook on one side for 3 to 4 minutes, until the edges become opaque. Squeeze the half lemon over the fish.

3. Flip the fish over, and cook on the other side for another 3 to 4 minutes.

4. Tilt the pan to gather the butter, and spoon it over the fish. Repeat a few times, and remove the pan from the heat.

5. Serve the fish with a sprinkle of parsley and a slice of lemon.

VARIATION 1 **LEMON-BUTTER TILAPIA WITH ALMONDS:** While the fish is cooking, toast ¼ cup slivered almonds in a dry pan until they begin to brown. Sprinkle the toasted almonds on the fish before serving.

VARIATION 2 **FISH PICCATA:** Add 2 tablespoons capers after cooking for more of a tangy taste.

PALEO PAIR: Serve with Roasted Broccoli with Lemon (page 135).

CEVICHE

Ceviche is one of the most delicious and refreshing dishes you'll ever enjoy. Basically, you "cook" raw fish in lemon or lime juice, which gives it a delectable flavor and smooth, delicate texture. When I was in Miami with my husband, we ate ceviche at least once a day; it reminded us of sushi, but with some fabulous Latin flair. **SERVES 4**

PREP TIME: 10 minutes, plus 6 hours to marinate
COOK TIME: None

1 pound halibut, diced

Juice of 2 large lemons

Juice of 4 limes

½ red onion, thinly sliced, divided

1 garlic clove, minced

1 jalapeño pepper, thinly sliced

Salt

Freshly ground black pepper

1 or 2 tablespoons sliced scallion, for garnish

1. In a large glass bowl, cover the diced fish with the lemon juice and lime juice. Stir, and add half the onion. Cover and refrigerate for 4 to 6 hours, or until the fish is completely opaque. Stir halfway through the marinating time to make sure the citrus is evenly "cooking" the fish.

2. Remove the fish from the refrigerator, drain, and discard the marinade. In a clean bowl, stir to combine the fish with the remaining onion, the garlic, and the jalapeño. Season with salt and pepper.

3. Spoon into serving dishes, top with the sliced scallion, and serve.

VARIATION 1 **SHRIMP CEVICHE:** Add a handful of precooked shrimp to the mix once it comes out of the refrigerator.

VARIATION 2 **ASIAN FUSION CEVICHE:** Follow the original recipe, and finish with a drizzle of sesame oil, a sprinkle of sesame seeds, and chopped fresh cilantro instead of the scallion.

PREP TIP: Unfortunately ceviche doesn't last very long in the refrigerator, so it's not something you can make ahead of time and serve later. To save time, cut up all your ingredients the night before.

SESAME MARINATED FISH

I'm not great at making and eating fish regularly, but I am a huge fan of Asian flavors, so this recipe is a tasty way to encourage myself to eat more seafood at home. The combination of sesame oil with fresh ginger and garlic is one of my favorites, and the coconut aminos adds a saltiness that brings the whole thing together. Then there's chili paste to add some heat, and a garnish of scallions for a pop of freshness right at the end. **SERVES 4**

PREP TIME: 5 minutes, plus 20 minutes to marinate
COOK TIME: 10 minutes

DP **NF**

1 tablespoon sesame oil

1 tablespoon fresh ginger, minced

1 teaspoon garlic, minced

1 teaspoon coconut aminos

1 teaspoon ground fresh chili paste

4 (6-ounce) white fish fillets (such as cod or halibut)

Freshly ground black pepper

1 to 2 tablespoons sliced scallions, for garnish

1. In a small bowl, stir to combine the sesame oil, ginger, garlic, coconut aminos, and chili paste. Using a brush, spread the marinade onto the fish. Marinate in the refrigerator for 20 minutes.

2. Remove the fish from the marinade (discard the marinade, although you can spoon a couple of tablespoons over the fish while it's cooking, if you like). In a large skillet over medium-high heat, cook the fish for about 5 minutes on each side, or until it turns white and begins to get flaky. Season with pepper.

3. Garnish with scallions and serve hot.

VARIATION 1 **SEARED TUNA STEAKS:** Use this marinade on thick tuna steaks, and sear them over high heat for 2 to 3 minutes on each side for medium-rare. Garnish with the scallions plus 1 or 2 tablespoons sesame seeds.

VARIATION 2 **WHITE FISH IN TOMATO SAUCE:** Heat 1½ cups tomato sauce (see page 22) in a large skillet, and place the fish on top. Cook for 4 to 5 minutes on each side. Spoon the sauce from the bottom of the pan on top of the fish, and garnish with ½ cup olives and a handful of chopped fresh parsley.

PALEO PAIR: Serve with Cauliflower Fried Rice (page 116) for a complete, Chinese-inspired dinner.

BAKED TILAPIA

Baked white fish is a great recipe to have when you're short on time but still want to serve a healthy and delicious meal. This recipe is your basic baked fish, and you can make it as is or experiment with some variations to come up with a truly unique dish perfect for your taste preferences. I love white fish with garlic, butter, and lots of lemon, so I generally don't stray from this recipe. **SERVES 4**

PREP TIME: 5 minutes
COOK TIME: 20 minutes

4 (6-ounce) pieces tilapia

Salt

Freshly ground black pepper

½ to 1 tablespoon garlic powder

¼ teaspoon red pepper flakes

4 tablespoons grass-fed butter

Juice of 1 lemon, plus 1 lemon cut into wedges

¼ cup chopped fresh parsley, for garnish

1. Preheat the oven to 400°F.

2. In an 8-by-12-inch baking dish, season the pieces of fish with salt, pepper, garlic powder, and red pepper flakes. Top with 1 tablespoon of butter on each piece of fish.

3. Bake for 15 minutes, or until the fish is white and opaque throughout.

4. Remove from the oven, and pour the lemon juice over the fish. Serve with a wedge of lemon and a sprinkle of parsley.

VARIATION 1 **BAKED SALMON:** Make this recipe with salmon if you're in the mood for a different kind of fish. The cook time may be a little longer. You can tell it's done when it flakes easily with a fork.

VARIATION 2 **BAKED TILAPIA WITH CAPERS AND HERBS:** Add 2 tablespoons capers and ¼ teaspoon each dried oregano, chives, and thyme to the fish before cooking.

PALEO PAIR: Serve with Squash Noodles in Walnut-Sage Butter (page 194).

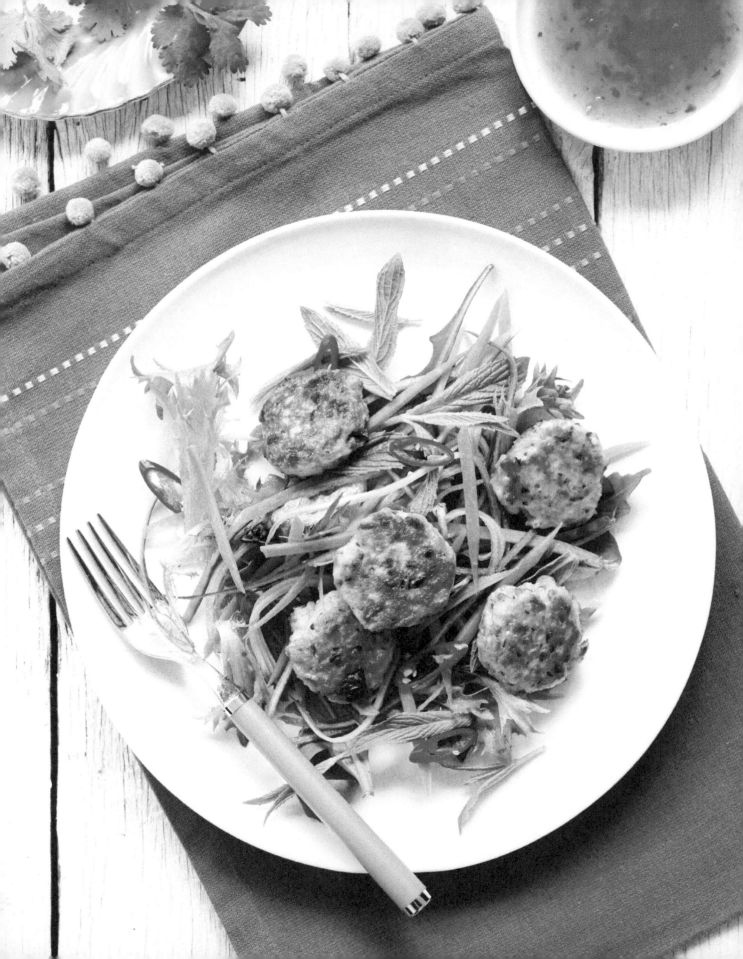

FISH CAKES

I'm always looking for new ways to serve fish, and these fish cakes are perfect. They're pretty easy to make and cook really fast, so you don't have to do a ton of prep work or spend a ton of time at the stove to make it happen. They're low-maintenance and really delicious. These work well as an appetizer, too—they're delicious with homemade spicy Paleo mayo, which I've included in the recipe below. **SERVES 4**

PREP TIME: 15 minutes
COOK TIME: 10 minutes

FOR THE FISH CAKES
2 (6-ounce) fillets white fish
2 tablespoons almond flour
1 large shallot, minced
¼ cup Homemade Mayo (page 47)
Zest of 1 lemon
Juice of ½ lemon
¼ cup minced fresh parsley
2 tablespoons Dijon mustard
1 large egg, slightly beaten
1 teaspoon ground paprika
Salt
Freshly ground black pepper
2 tablespoons extra-virgin olive oil

FOR THE CHILI SAUCE
2 tablespoons hot chili oil
¼ cup apple cider vinegar
¼ cup olive oil

TO SERVE
½ cup mizuna (or other lettuce)
½ cup arugula
1 carrot, julienned
1 small red chile, sliced

1. Chop the fish into a fine mince, and place in a large bowl.

2. Add the almond flour, shallot, Homemade Mayo, lemon zest and juice, parsley, mustard, egg, paprika, salt, and pepper, and mix well. Shape the mixture into four large cakes or eight smaller ones (smaller will be easier to turn over when cooking).

3. In a large nonstick sauté pan over medium-high heat, heat the olive oil. Add the fish cakes, and allow them to brown, 4 to 5 minutes. Gently flip each one, reshaping as needed, and brown the other side, 4 to 5 minutes more.

4. For the chili sauce, combine all ingredients in a small bowl.

5. To serve, layer greens, carrot, and chiles on serving plates, and top with fish cakes and chili sauce as desired.

VARIATION 1 **CRAB CAKES:** Replace the fish with crab, and follow the recipe as written. Crab is less flaky and has a stronger seafood flavor than milder white fish.

VARIATION 2 **SALMON CAKES:** Replace the white fish with 2 (6-ounce) cans salmon. Drain the salmon, follow the original recipe as written, and enjoy the hit of heart-healthy fats.

PALEO PAIR: Serve with Broccoli Slaw (page 134).

CITRUS-BAKED FISH

I think grilling is my favorite way to cook fish, but baking comes in a close second. It takes no time at all and uses minimal dishes, which I love when it's time to clean up. This citrusy fish is fresh, fast, and delicious. Topped with lots of fresh herbs, it makes for a delightful light lunch when it's hot outside. **SERVES 4**

PREP TIME: 10 minutes
COOK TIME: 15 minutes

30 **DF** **NF**

2 lemons, sliced, divided

3 limes, sliced, divided

4 to 6 (6-ounce) fillets white fish (such as cod)

Salt

Freshly ground black pepper

1 tablespoon chopped fresh dill

1 tablespoon chopped fresh parsley

1. Preheat the oven to 400°F.

2. In an 8-by-12-inch baking dish, layer half of the sliced lemons and limes to cover the bottom of the pan. Top with the fish fillets, and season with salt and pepper.

3. Layer the remaining lemon and lime slices on top, and bake for 10 to 15 minutes, until the fish flakes easily with a fork.

4. Remove from the oven, and serve the fish topped with the dill and parsley.

VARIATION 1 **CITRUS-BAKED FISH WITH ORANGES:** Swap out the lemons (or limes, whichever you prefer) for oranges for a sweeter version.

VARIATION 2 **CITRUS-BAKED SALMON:** Use salmon instead of white fish. The cook time may be a little longer—check them after 10 minutes. You'll know it's done when it flakes easily with a fork. Salmon is loaded with healthy fats, so it's a great alternative.

PREP TIP: Layer up the dish ahead of time, and pop it in the oven before dinner.

POACHED FISH WITH VEGETABLES

This is an easily prepared, simple, comforting fish recipe that always tastes great. It starts with a basic medley of vegetables known as mirepoix (2 parts onion, 1 part celery, 1 part carrot). I like to make this recipe with a thinner cut of fish because it cooks a lot faster, but with this cooking method, the possibilities really are endless. **SERVES 2**

PREP TIME: 10 minutes
COOK TIME: 15 minutes

2 tablespoons grass-fed butter

2 (6-ounce) pieces white fish (such as cod or halibut)

½ cup diced onion

¼ cup diced carrot

¼ cup diced celery

2 or 3 fresh thyme sprigs, plus an extra pinch for garnish

1 large rosemary sprig, plus an extra pinch for garnish

2 or 3 fresh sage leaves (or pinch dried)

1 cup vegetable broth

Salt

Freshly ground black pepper

1. In a large skillet over medium-high heat, melt the butter. Quickly sear the fish, about 1 minute on each side. Remove it from the pan, and add the onion, carrot, celery, thyme, rosemary, and sage to the pan. Stir and sauté for 5 minutes.

2. Pour the vegetable broth into the skillet, and bring to a simmer. Return the fish to the skillet, and slowly poach until cooked throughout, 5 to 7 minutes.

3. Season with salt and pepper, and serve garnished with more fresh herbs.

VARIATION 1 **POACHED TUNA STEAKS:** Make this recipe with thick steaks of tuna instead. Follow the original recipe, but allow a few minutes more cooking time (tuna is delicious rare or medium-rare, so don't overcook it).

VARIATION 2 **SUMMER VEGGIE POACHED FISH:** Add more vegetables to the original recipe—1 diced zucchini, 1 diced squash, and 1 cup cherry tomatoes, halved. Put them in the pan after you've sautéed the onion, carrot, and celery, and allow to cook for 5 to 7 minutes before adding the fish back in.

PREP TIP: Mirepoix is the base for a huge number of soups and stews, and you can make it very easily ahead of time so you don't have to spend 10 to 15 minutes chopping when it's time to cook. You can store it in a container in the refrigerator for up to 3 days so you'll always have it on hand.

MAHI MAHI WITH MANGO-PEACH SALSA

I love grilled white fish with a fruity salsa, and this easy mahi mahi topped with mango and peach is definitely a favorite. It's perfect for warmer days, and you can make a bunch of the salsa and leave it in the refrigerator for leftovers—it does great after a few days of marinating. If you don't have access to a grill, you can easily cook the fish inside on a grill pan or just in a regular skillet. **SERVES 4**

PREP TIME: 15 minutes
COOK TIME: 10 minutes

FOR THE MANGO-PEACH SALSA

1 avocado, diced

1 mango, diced

1 peach, diced

½ pineapple, diced

½ red onion, minced

Juice of 1 lime

1 bunch fresh cilantro, chopped

¼ teaspoon ground cayenne pepper

FOR THE FISH

4 (6-ounce) pieces mahi mahi

1 to 2 tablespoons extra-virgin olive oil

Salt

Freshly ground black pepper

Chopped fresh cilantro, for garnish

1 or 2 limes, quartered

TO MAKE THE MANGO-PEACH SALSA

In a large bowl, mix the avocado, mango, peach, pineapple, red onion, lime juice, cilantro, and cayenne. Cover with plastic wrap, and refrigerate until ready to serve.

TO MAKE THE FISH

1. Preheat the grill to medium-high.

2. Coat the fish with the olive oil, and season with salt and pepper. Grill for 3 to 4 minutes per side, until the fish is opaque all the way through.

3. Serve the fish hot with a couple of tablespoons of the salsa on top or on the side. Garnish with extra cilantro and a wedge of lime.

VARIATION 1 **BLACKENED MAHI MAHI:** Season the mahi mahi with Blackening Spice Mix (page 161), and cook in a dry pan for 3 to 4 minutes per side.

VARIATION 2 **SEA BASS WITH MANGO SALSA:** Substitute mahi mahi for sea bass if you're interested in a flakier, more buttery white fish. Cook for 6 to 7 minutes per side, until opaque all the way through.

PREP TIP: Buying mahi mahi frozen at the store is so convenient—it keeps really well in the freezer and can be defrosted overnight to be ready to cook for dinner the next day. If you forget to take it out of the freezer in time, you can actually defrost it even more quickly in the sink!

FISH STEW

I absolutely love a hearty fish stew. It always makes me think about the Italian side of my family, gathered around the table, probably on Christmas Eve, when my grandfather would traditionally make fish. The bacon gives this stew a beautiful depth of flavor, and the crushed tomatoes melding with the chicken broth to lightly poach the seafood produces a lovely aroma. Comfort food at its finest. **SERVES 4 TO 6**

PREP TIME: 15 minutes
COOK TIME: 25 minutes

5 shallots, sliced

4 slices bacon, diced

3 garlic cloves, minced

½ cup white wine (optional; omit if strict Paleo)

1½ cups chicken broth

1 (28-ounce) can crushed tomatoes

20 small scallops

12 ounces white fish (such as haddock)

Salt

Freshly ground black pepper

1. In a large saucepan over medium heat, sauté the shallots, bacon, and garlic for 7 to 10 minutes, until the bacon is crisp.

2. Pour in the wine or a splash of the chicken broth, and deglaze the pan, stirring to scrape up the browned bits from the bottom.

3. Add the broth and tomatoes to the pot, and cook for another 5 minutes.

4. Gently add the scallops and fish, and cook for 5 to 10 minutes more, or until all the seafood is opaque and cooked through.

5. Season with salt and pepper, and serve.

VARIATION 1 **FISH STEW WITH VEGETABLES:** After sautéing the shallots, bacon, and garlic, add 2 chopped celery stalks, 3 or 4 chopped carrots, and 1 diced zucchini to the pan. Cook for 5 to 7 minutes before continuing with the recipe as written from step 2.

VARIATION 2 **FISH STEW WITH MUSSELS:** Soak ½ pound mussels in cold water for about 15 minutes. Scrub them with a vegetable brush, and discard any that are already open. Add them to the stew with the scallops and fish in step 4, and cook for 10 minutes. Discard any that don't open.

PALEO PAIR: Serve with Roasted Broccoli with Lemon (page 135).

SEA BASS TOPPED WITH CRAB

If you've ever seen Chilean sea bass as a special on a menu somewhere, chances are the server has talked it up. Sea bass is super delicious and has one of the best textures around, with moist, thick, buttery but still flaky flesh that holds up to a variety of flavors and cooking methods. You can often find it stuffed or topped with crab, like in this recipe.

Fun fact: Chilean sea bass used to be known as Patagonian Tooth Fish until a fish wholesaler in 1977 rebranded it to sound fancier. Since then, it's only risen in popularity. Whatever its true name, I just call it wonderful. **SERVES 4**

PREP TIME: 5 minutes
COOK TIME: 10 minutes

1 tablespoon extra-virgin olive oil

4 (6-ounce) pieces sea bass

8 ounces crab meat, drained

1 tablespoon freshly squeezed lemon juice

1 teaspoon chopped fresh thyme leaves

Salt

Freshly ground black pepper

1 or 2 tablespoons sliced scallion, for garnish

1. In a large skillet over medium-high heat, heat the olive oil. Fry the sea bass for about 3 minutes, then turn it, keeping the whole piece intact. Cook for an additional 3 minutes on the other side.

2. In a small bowl, mix the crab meat with the lemon juice and thyme. Season with salt and pepper.

3. Plate the fish, and serve topped with the crab meat and garnished with the sliced scallions.

VARIATION 1 **SCALLOPS TOPPED WITH CRAB:** Instead of fish, quickly sauté 10 to 20 small scallops (or 5 to 10 larger ones) in hot butter over medium-high heat for 1½ to 2 minutes per side, depending on their size. The delicately sweet flesh caramelizes beautifully.

VARIATION 2 **SEA BASS TOPPED WITH CRAB AND PINEAPPLE CURRY SAUCE:** In a saucepan, whisk ¼ cup pineapple juice, 1½ teaspoons curry powder, ½ teaspoon ginger, the juice of 1 lime, and 2 to 3 tablespoons canned coconut cream (the solid part that sits on top of coconut milk when refrigerated). Bring to a gentle boil, and then reduce the heat to low and simmer until thick. Pour over the crab-topped sea bass and serve hot with an extra wedge of lime.

PALEO PAIR: Serve with Squash Noodles in Walnut-Sage Butter (page 194).

PANTRY BASIC: BALSAMIC VINAIGRETTE

If I make a salad and I'm not feeling creative, I'll just dress it with balsamic vinaigrette—it's good on everything, and it's super easy to make. Sometimes I like to add herbs like chopped basil, but this basic recipe is a really solid one as is.

MAKES 1½ CUPS

PREP TIME: 5 minutes
COOK TIME: None

`30` `NF` `V`

1 cup extra-virgin olive oil

½ cup balsamic vinegar

1 garlic clove, minced

1 tablespoon Dijon mustard

Pinch salt

Pinch freshly ground
black pepper

1. In a mason jar or other container with a tightly fitting lid, shake or mix well to combine the olive oil, vinegar, garlic, Dijon mustard, salt, and pepper.

2. Store refrigerated, and take it out 20 minutes before using, since the dressing will need time to come to room temperature.

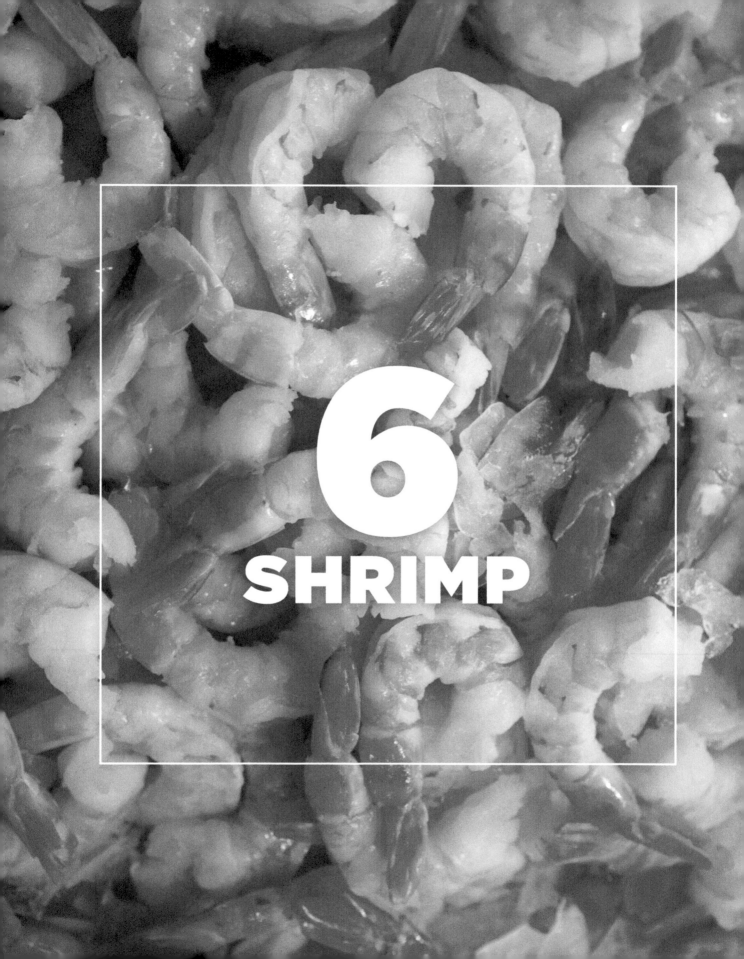

6
SHRIMP

Whether you're making an appetizer or a main course, shrimp is always a good choice. Here you have recipes for both, like Bacon-Wrapped Shrimp (page 92), which will always be a huge hit at a party, or the easy one-pot Shrimp Stir-Fry (page 96) that you could make for dinner tonight, as well as a few that could go either way or be great light lunches. Blackened Shrimp Tacos (page 93), anyone?

In most of the recipes, I've made a note of whether you should keep the tails on or off, but you can keep them on (and even leave the shell on) if you prefer it that way. There's just something about the look and feel of peeling my own shrimp that I really like, so a lot of the time I'll sauté them unpeeled and serve them that way—it really just depends on the dish. For example, finger foods like tacos are definitely better without the shells on, while paella is traditionally served with shells.

BACON-WRAPPED SHRIMP

I am a bit notorious among my family and friends for wanting to wrap everything in bacon. Avocados, sweet potatoes, dates—you name it, I've probably wrapped it in bacon at some point, so this bacon-wrapped shrimp recipe was really only a matter of time. The combination of sweet shrimp and salty bacon is a surefire winner, making these great to serve as an appetizer with a little sweet chili oil on the side for dipping; they really go with almost any main course you choose! **SERVES 4**

PREP TIME: 10 minutes
COOK TIME: 10 minutes

1 pound shrimp, peeled and deveined (you can leave the tails on)

12 slices bacon, halved, plus more if necessary

Chopped fresh parsley, for garnish

1. Preheat the oven to 400°F.

2. Wrap a piece of bacon around each shrimp, and line them up on a baking sheet. Bake for 8 to 10 minutes, or until the bacon is crispy.

3. Remove from the oven and serve hot on a platter, sprinkled with parsley.

VARIATION 1 **GRILLED BACON-WRAPPED SHRIMP KEBABS:** Use skewers to hold the shrimp in place, and grill for 5 to 6 minutes on each side instead of cooking them in the oven. Finish with a squeeze of fresh lime juice.

VARIATION 2 **MARINATED BACON-WRAPPED SHRIMP:** Before wrapping the shrimp with bacon, marinate them in a mixture of ¼ cup extra-virgin olive oil, ¼ cup red wine vinegar, 1 chopped garlic clove, and 1 tablespoon of an Asian chili paste.

PALEO PAIR: Turn this appetizer into lunch or dinner with a side of Kale Salad with Onion and Avocado (page 128).

BLACKENED SHRIMP TACOS

When it comes to non-Paleo food, my favorites are Asian and Mexican. It's hard for me to resist a taco, so when I find a place that offers lettuce cups instead of tortillas, I feel like I've won the lottery. That's how I make them at home, and it's refreshing and just as tasty as a flour or corn tortilla. These blackened shrimp tacos are spicy and juicy and so great served over a crispy lettuce leaf with a squeeze of lime. **SERVES 4**

PREP TIME: 10 minutes
COOK TIME: 10 minutes

1½ pounds shrimp, peeled and deveined

2 tablespoons extra-virgin olive oil, divided

2 to 3 tablespoons Blackening Spice Mix (page 161)

8 lettuce cups, either romaine leaves or butter lettuce

4 tablespoons salsa

1 avocado, cut into slices

1 lime, cut into wedges

3 to 4 tablespoons chopped fresh cilantro, for garnish

1. In a large bowl, drizzle the shrimp with 1 tablespoon of olive oil, and add the Blackening Spice Mix. Use your hands to thoroughly mix until all the shrimp are coated with seasoning.

2. In a large pan over medium heat, heat the remaining 1 tablespoon of olive oil. Add the shrimp, and stir quickly until pink, 5 to 7 minutes.

3. Serve the shrimp in the lettuce cups, topped with the salsa, sliced avocado, and a wedge of lime and garnished with the cilantro.

VARIATION 1 **SALT AND PEPPER SHRIMP TACOS:** If you aren't in the mood for spicy blackened shrimp, skip the Blackening Spice Mix and simply season with salt and pepper. Follow the original recipe as written.

VARIATION 2 **ASIAN SHRIMP TACOS:** Instead of olive oil, season the shrimp with 1 tablespoon sesame oil and 1 tablespoon freshly grated ginger. Cook the shrimp according to the original recipe, and swap out the original toppings for 1 tablespoon each shredded carrots and cucumber. Keep the cilantro for garnish.

PALEO PAIR: Serve with a side of fresh guacamole (see page 37).

THAI SHRIMP SALAD

A Thai-inspired shrimp salad has got to be one of the most refreshing and satisfying meals out there. When you order it in a restaurant, the dressing tends to be loaded with sugar, so I made this Paleo-friendly version for when I'm hit with a Thai craving (a fairly frequent occurrence for me!), but don't want to indulge in hidden sugars. **SERVES 4**

PREP TIME: 10 minutes
COOK TIME: None

2 garlic cloves, minced

2 or 3 scallions, chopped

¼ cup freshly squeezed lime juice (3 or 4 limes)

2 tablespoons fish sauce

¼ teaspoon chili powder

Salt

Freshly ground black pepper

2 cups chopped romaine lettuce

1½ pounds cooked, chilled shrimp, peeled and deveined

½ red onion, thinly sliced

¼ cup cherry tomatoes, chopped

1 large cucumber, julienned

5 to 10 fresh mint leaves, chopped

1 small bunch fresh cilantro, chopped

1. In a small bowl, mix the garlic, scallions, lime juice, fish sauce, and chili powder, and season with salt and pepper.

2. In a large bowl, layer the chopped romaine and shrimp. Add the onion, tomatoes, and cucumber. Pour the dressing over the salad, and toss well. Top with the mint and cilantro, and serve immediately.

VARIATION 1 **SHRIMP SALAD WITH AVOCADO:** Add some healthy fats to your salad by topping it with a diced avocado. Squeeze a lemon over it to prevent the avocado from browning.

VARIATION 2 **THAI CRAB SALAD:** Replace the shrimp with canned crab for a stronger flavor.

PREP TIP: Buy precooked frozen shrimp, and defrost them while you assemble the salad and dressing.

SHRIMP SALAD WITH TOMATO AND LEMON

When I was first learning to cook for myself, one of my favorite recipes was a shrimp and orzo salad with feta cheese that was served at room temperature, kind of—the pasta was warm and the shrimp was cold, and it was just really satisfying on many levels. This recipe is inspired by that one, although you won't find pasta or cheese here. What I held on to, though, was the bright tomatoes, lots of lemon juice, and parsley that make this dish so perfect to eat outside on a warm afternoon. **SERVES 4**

PREP TIME: 10 minutes
COOK TIME: None

1½ to 2 pounds cooked shrimp, chilled

10 ounces cherry tomatoes, at room temperature (don't refrigerate at all)

2 garlic cloves, minced

½ red onion, thinly sliced

Juice of 2 lemons

2 tablespoons extra-virgin olive oil

Salt

Freshly ground black pepper

¼ cup fresh parsley, chopped

1. In a large bowl, mix well to combine the shrimp, tomatoes, garlic, red onion, lemon juice, and olive oil. Season with salt and pepper.

2. Serve right away, topped with the fresh parsley.

VARIATION 1 **SHRIMP AND TOMATO SALAD WITH AVOCADO:** Add 1 or 2 diced avocados to the salad. You may need to add more salt and pepper.

VARIATION 2 **CRAB SALAD WITH TOMATO AND LEMON:** Switch the shrimp for crab—fresh or canned work equally well. Crab is also sweet but more strongly flavored than shrimp.

PALEO PAIR: Serve with a side of Roasted Broccoli with Lemon (page 135).

SHRIMP STIR-FRY

Stir-fries were never my favorite as a kid—something about the large quantity of vegetables didn't sit right with me, and I disliked cooked green bell peppers, which usually play a key role. But my palate changed as I grew up, and when I started cooking for myself I became more and more a fan of one-pot dishes. The trick is to get the vegetables hot enough so they get nice and caramelized. The other trick is butter. **SERVES 4**

PREP TIME: 10 minutes
COOK TIME: 20 minutes

2 tablespoons grass-fed butter

½ onion, diced

2 garlic cloves, minced

1 green bell pepper, cut into strips

1 pound shrimp, peeled and deveined

½ cup cherry tomatoes

1 tablespoon sesame oil

1 tablespoon sesame seeds, for garnish

1 to 2 tablespoons sliced scallions, for garnish

1. In a large skillet over medium heat, melt the butter. Sauté the onion until slightly translucent, about 5 minutes. Add the garlic and bell pepper, and cook for another 5 to 7 minutes.

2. Add the shrimp, and cook until pink, about 5 minutes. Throw in the cherry tomatoes, and stir them around for another 3 to 5 minutes, or until a few of them start to burst. Continuing to stir, drizzle the sesame oil over everything as you turn off the heat.

3. Serve the stir-fry hot, topped with the sesame seeds and scallions.

VARIATION 1 **SURF AND TURF STIR-FRY:** Add 6 to 8 ounces sliced steak to the stir-fry. Cook for a few minutes before adding the shrimp, or if you have some already cooked, just throw them in to heat up with the tomatoes.

VARIATION 2 **CHICKEN STIR-FRY:** Switch things up by using diced chicken breast instead of shrimp. Depending on the size of the pieces, you'll need to let it cook for an additional 5 to 7 minutes.

PALEO PAIR: Serve with a side of Cauliflower Fried Rice (page 116).

COCONUT SHRIMP

One of my husband's favorite dishes is coconut shrimp, but I rarely make it for him at home because it's usually battered and fried. I remember the first time he ordered it—I think we were at an Outback Steakhouse—and I found it strange (in a really charming way): Here's a dish that I don't ever think about, and it's one of his favorites. Getting to know someone is fascinating. Here's my recipe for Paleo coconut shrimp, which I make for my husband whenever I think about that date we had back in college. **SERVES 4**

PREP TIME: 10 minutes
COOK TIME: 15 minutes

2 to 3 pounds shrimp, peeled and deveined, tails on

2 eggs, whisked

1 tablespoon tapioca starch

1 cup shredded unsweetened coconut

Salt

Freshly ground black pepper

1 tablespoon coconut oil

1. Butterfly the shrimp by slicing them down the back so they open a bit.

2. In a small bowl, whisk the egg and tapioca starch together. Pour the coconut into another small bowl. Dip the shrimp into the egg mixture. Let any excess drip off, and then dip them into the coconut to coat them. Season with salt and pepper.

3. In a large skillet over medium heat, heat the coconut oil. Working in batches so you don't crowd the pan, fry the shrimp for 3 to 5 minutes, or until they are pink and the coconut is lightly browned. Keep cooked shrimp warm by placing them in an ovenproof dish and into a 200°F oven.

4. Serve immediately.

VARIATION 1 COCONUT SHRIMP WITH MANGO SAUCE: Make the apricot sauce (see page 73) with mangos instead of apricot for a sweeter result. Pour the sauce into a ramekin or small dish, and serve alongside the coconut shrimp.

VARIATION 2 COCONUT SHRIMP WITH COCKTAIL SAUCE: Mix half of a 14.5-ounce can diced tomatoes with 2 tablespoons tomato paste, ¼ cup horseradish, and the juice of half a lemon. Season with salt and pepper, and serve with the shrimp.

PALEO PAIR: Serve with a side of Beet Chips (page 173) and a scoop of Mango-Peach Salsa (page 86).

SHRIMP KEBABS

My brother and I made kebabs for our dad one Father's Day—it seemed like the perfect summer Sunday dinner. They take a little time to put together, but they cook super fast, especially when using shrimp. I love making kebabs for a party because I usually have someone with me in the kitchen (usually my brother). Meal prep is always better with a buddy. **SERVES 4 TO 6**

PREP TIME: 15 minutes
COOK TIME: 15 minutes

1 pound raw shrimp, peeled and deveined

1 red onion, quartered and separated into layers

1 large zucchini, quartered and diced

½ pound salmon

1 to 2 tablespoons extra-virgin olive oil

½ tablespoon garlic powder

Salt

Freshly ground black pepper

1. Preheat the grill to medium-high heat.

2. On a baking sheet, lay out the shrimp, onion, and zucchini. Carefully spear a piece of shrimp, a piece of onion, a piece of zucchini, and piece of salmon onto a kebab skewer. Repeat until the skewer is almost full. Repeat with the remaining skewers until the ingredients are all used.

3. Drizzle some olive oil evenly over the kebabs, and season with the garlic powder, salt, and pepper. Grill (or sauté in a large skillet over medium-high heat) for 5 to 7 minutes on each side, or until the shrimp are pink and the veggies are tender.

4. Use a fork or tongs to slide the kebabs off the spears, and serve hot.

VARIATION 1 **BBQ SHRIMP KEBABS:** Brush the kebabs with BBQ Sauce (page 131) before cooking.

VARIATION 2 **CHICKEN, STEAK, AND SHRIMP KEBABS:** Add more protein to your kebabs with diced chicken breast and diced steak (a thin, cheaper cut will do just fine). Make sure the chicken is done before removing it from the heat—cut it into smaller pieces so you don't overcook the shrimp and beef.

PREP TIP: Assemble the kebabs a day or two ahead of time so all you'll have to do is cook them when it's time to eat.

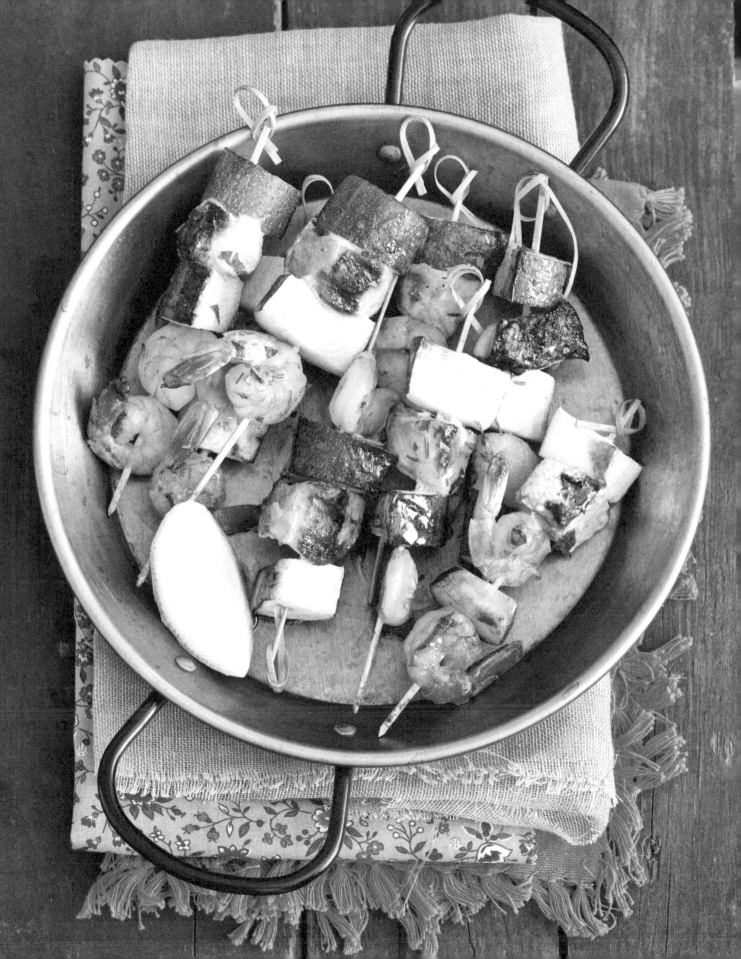

GREEN SHRIMP

I love this recipe because even though the flavors are super vibrant and strong, the shrimp itself is really versatile and can be added to a great number of meals. I love these "green shrimp" in the spring and summer with a squeeze of lemon—the herby marinade makes for a refreshing warm-weather dinner!

SERVES 2

PREP TIME: 10 minutes, plus 1 hour to marinate
COOK TIME: 10 minutes

½ cup chopped fresh basil

½ cup chopped fresh parsley

2 garlic cloves, minced

¼ cup extra-virgin olive oil

1½ pounds raw shrimp, shelled and deveined

Salt

Freshly ground black pepper

1. In a large bowl, stir to combine the basil, parsley, garlic, and olive oil. Add the shrimp, season with salt and pepper, and mix until the shrimp are covered with the marinade. Marinate in the refrigerator for at least 1 hour.

2. Preheat the grill (or a large skillet on the stove) to medium-high heat.

3. Grill (or sauté) the shrimp until pink, about 3 to 4 minutes on each side, and serve.

VARIATION 1 **GREEN SHRIMP SALAD:** Add ½ diced tomato, 6 to 8 chopped pepperoncini, and 5 chopped sun-dried tomatoes to the green shrimp. Stir in about ½ cup Homemade Mayo (page 47), and season with salt and pepper.

VARIATION 2 **GREEN CHICKEN:** Use this herbaceous marinade on chicken! Marinate 1½ pounds chicken breast or thighs (cut into chunks), and cook for 7 to 10 minutes, until browned and cooked through.

PALEO PAIR: This shrimp is lovely on a salad with fresh greens, diced mango, and a drizzle of the green marinade in the recipe. Just make a fresh batch—never reuse any marinades that have touched raw meat.

PAELLA

If you've ever had paella, then you know how complex and savory the flavors are. It's a Spanish rice dish usually infused with saffron and loaded with lots of seafood and sometimes meat. Because the rice is arguably the main ingredient, a Paleo paella might seem a little counterintuitive, but this one has many of the same spices (including saffron, which gives paella its gorgeous color), as well as the more typical shrimp, chicken, and sausage. **SERVES 6**

PREP TIME: 15 minutes
COOK TIME: 1 hour, 40 minutes

1 large onion, sliced

1 tablespoon extra-virgin olive oil

Salt

Freshly ground black pepper

1 head garlic

1 pound asparagus, cut into 1-inch pieces

1 pound Italian sausage

1 pound boneless chicken breast, diced

1 teaspoon ground paprika

½ cup white wine (optional; omit if strict Paleo)

1½ cups chicken broth

2 pounds raw shrimp, peeled and deveined

Pinch saffron threads

1. Preheat the oven to 450°F.

2. On a baking sheet, sprinkle the onion with the olive oil, and season with salt and pepper. Cut the top off the head of garlic, remove the outer papery skin, and wrap the head in aluminum foil. Roast the onion and garlic for 20 minutes.

3. Transfer the cooked onion to a large bowl, leaving the garlic on the baking sheet. Put the asparagus on the baking sheet with the garlic, and roast them together for 10 minutes more. Remove the asparagus from the oven, and add to the bowl with the onion. Return the garlic to the oven to roast alone for 10 more minutes.

4. In a large skillet over medium-high heat, cook the sausage until the whole outside is browned, 5 to 7 minutes per side. Remove, slice, and return to the skillet. Continue to cook, flipping and stirring, until browned inside, 5 to 7 minutes more. Remove it from the skillet, and put it in the bowl with the onion and asparagus.

5. Sauté the chicken in the sausage fat until the outsides are browned, 7 to 10 minutes. Add the paprika, and season with salt and pepper.

6. Pour in the wine or some chicken broth and deglaze the pan, stirring to scrape up any browned bits, and then add the rest of the chicken broth. Reduce the heat to low, and simmer for 30 minutes. ❯

PREP TIP: You can cook all the ingredients ahead of time and throw them together 30 minutes before you're ready to serve it.

7. Add the shrimp and the roasted garlic. Stir and cook until the shrimp are pink, about 5 minutes, and then return the onion, asparagus, sausage, and chicken to the skillet. Add the saffron, and continue to cook on low until ready to serve.

VARIATION 1 **PAELLA WITH CAULIFLOWER RICE:** Since traditional paella is cooked with rice, you can create a more authentic, but still Paleo, version of the dish by serving this on top of a bed of Plain Cauliflower Rice (page 116).

VARIATION 2 **LOBSTER PAELLA:** Make this paella extra special by serving it topped with lobster tails, steamed in an inch or two of water for about 8 minutes.

SHRIMP GUMBO

When I think of gumbo, I usually think of rice, so for a long time I didn't make it—but gumbo itself is actually very Paleo-friendly. Traditional gumbos start with a roux, which includes flour, but I skip it completely and am always really happy with the consistency. If you like it a little thicker (or with more liquid), you can adjust the amount of chicken broth. This shrimp gumbo is spicy and delicious, whether it's Mardi Gras or not. **SERVES 4 TO 6**

PREP TIME: 10 minutes
COOK TIME: 40 minutes

2 tablespoons extra-virgin olive oil

1 onion, diced

½ green bell pepper, diced

½ red bell pepper, diced

2 celery stalks, diced

2 tablespoons Cajun seasoning

1 (14.5-ounce) can diced tomatoes, drained

½ cup chicken broth

2 dried bay leaves

1 pound raw shrimp, shells on

Salt

Freshly ground black pepper

Chopped fresh parsley, for garnish

1. In a large pot or Dutch oven over medium heat, heat the olive oil. Sauté the onion, green and red bell peppers, celery, and Cajun seasoning for 5 to 7 minutes.

2. Add the tomatoes to the pot, and stir well. Add the chicken broth and bay leaves, and bring to a boil. Reduce the heat to low, and simmer for at least 30 minutes.

3. Season the shrimp with salt and pepper, and add them to the pot 5 minutes before serving. When the shrimp are pink, serve the gumbo in bowls garnished with parsley.

VARIATION 1 **SHRIMP AND SAUSAGE GUMBO:** Make this gumbo spicier and a bit heartier by adding sausage. Cook 1 pound andouille sausage in a pan for 5 to 7 minutes, until browned, and allow to cool before cutting into ½-inch slices. Add the slices to the pot with the tomatoes.

VARIATION 2 **CHICKEN GUMBO:** This recipe works really well using 2 pounds diced chicken instead of the shrimp, so if that's what you have in your refrigerator, don't hold back. The chicken may take longer to cook, depending on the size of the dice, so make sure it's cooked through.

PALEO PAIR: Serve with a side of Plain Cauliflower Rice (page 116).

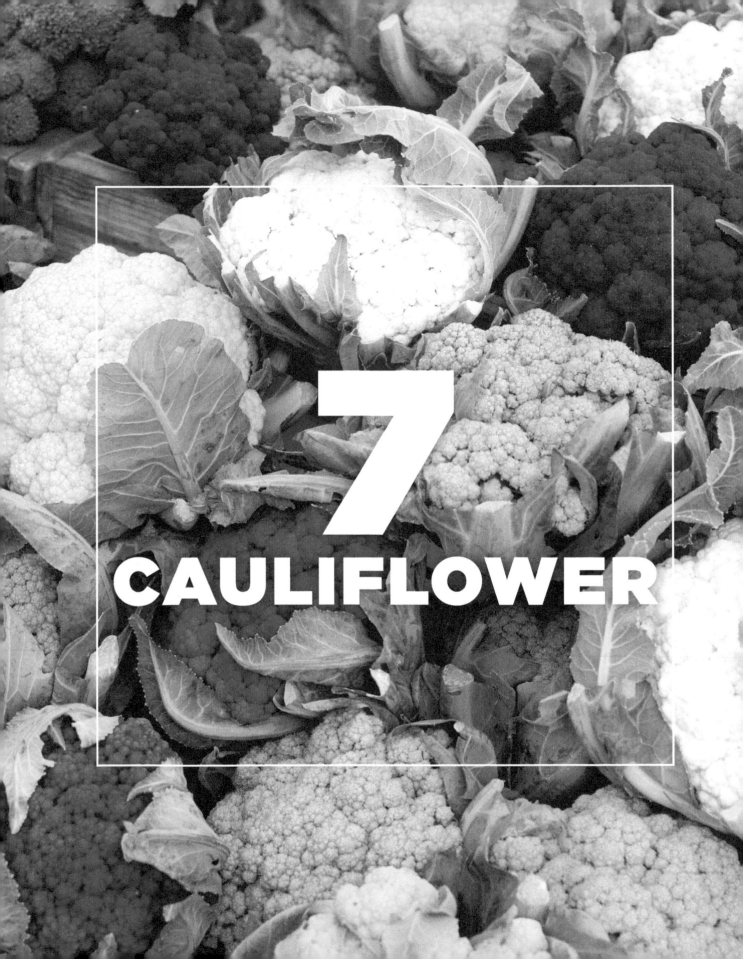

7
CAULIFLOWER

Cauliflower is one of the most popular vegetables in the Paleo community because you can do so much with it to replace grains and carbs. It makes a great substitute for rice if you throw it in a food processor and then sauté it, and you can even make pizza crust, tortillas, and a lot more.

For this book we wanted to stick with straightforward recipes that don't call for a ton of time or ingredients, so I skipped pizza crust and stuck with some of my favorite mashed and roasted cauliflower recipes—although I couldn't resist including one for Cauliflower Risotto (page 107) and my favorite cauliflower recipe of all time, Cauliflower Fried Rice (page 116).

There are so many things you can do with a simple head of cauliflower, and I'm excited to share ten of my favorites with you. I hope they inspire you to branch out and get creative with this versatile vegetable.

GARLIC-ROASTED MASHED CAULIFLOWER

I really believe that you could make a great batch of mashed cauliflower and serve it to someone without mentioning what it is, and they would probably assume it was mashed potatoes—that's how awesome cauliflower is. You can boil it and then mash it the way you would with potatoes, but for this recipe we first roast it with garlic to get some beautiful browning action. Then it goes into a bowl with butter and some chicken broth before being blended into the most comforting of side dishes. **SERVES 4**

PREP TIME: 10 minutes
COOK TIME: 45 minutes

NF

1 large head cauliflower, cut into florets

1 to 2 tablespoons extra-virgin olive oil

Salt

Freshly ground black pepper

½ head garlic

¼ cup chicken broth, plus more if necessary

2 to 3 tablespoons grass-fed butter

1. Preheat the oven to 400°F.

2. On a large baking sheet, spread out the cauliflower florets, and drizzle with the olive oil. Season with salt and pepper, and mix it all up with your hands. Slice the top off the head of garlic, and peel the outer skin off to leave the cloves exposed. Wrap the garlic with aluminum foil before placing it on the baking sheet with the cauliflower. Bake for 30 to 40 minutes, or until the cauliflower begins to brown. Remove from the oven.

3. Meanwhile, in a large saucepan over medium heat, warm the chicken broth. Transfer the cauliflower and roasted garlic to the saucepan, and carefully blend with an immersion blender or hand mixer. If it's too dry, add another splash or two of chicken broth.

4. Add the butter, and mix it in until melted. Season with salt and pepper, and serve.

VARIATION 1 **TRUFFLE MASHED CAULIFLOWER:** Prepare the mashed cauliflower according to the original recipe, and add a tiny drizzle of truffle oil (no more than ¼ or ½ teaspoon) once you've removed the pan from the heat. Truffle oil is expensive, but it's super strong, so you only need a tiny bit; even a small bottle will last a long time.

VARIATION 2 **NON-ROASTED MASHED CAULIFLOWER:** Instead of roasting the cauliflower, cook it in boiling water for 10 to 12 minutes, or until fork-tender. Drain and return it to the pan, where you'll continue with the recipe as written (minus the garlic).

PALEO PAIR: This makes a delicious side dish for Beef Tenderloin (page 56).

CAULIFLOWER RISOTTO

This faux-sotto, made with riced cauliflower, is a lot quicker than traditional risotto because there are no grains to cook down, which makes it both easier and more challenging. It's easier because it's fast, but it's a bit more challenging to achieve a risotto-like consistency without rice or cream. Cauliflower is extremely hardy and versatile, though, so with the help of shallots, mushrooms, and some butter, we get pretty darn close. **SERVES 4**

PREP TIME: 10 minutes
COOK TIME: 20 minutes

2 heads cauliflower, cut into florets

2 tablespoons grass-fed butter

10 ounces mushrooms, sliced

1 garlic clove, minced

1 shallot, minced

¼ cup white wine (or chicken broth if strict Paleo)

1½ cups chicken broth

1 to 2 tablespoons sliced scallions

1. In a food processor or blender, roughly chop the cauliflower florets. You want it to be the consistency of regular rice.

2. In a large pan over medium heat, melt the butter. Sauté the mushrooms, garlic, and shallot for about 5 minutes, or until the shallot becomes translucent. Add the cauliflower, and continue to sauté for another 5 to 7 minutes.

3. Pour in the wine or broth, and deglaze the pan, stirring to scrape up the browned bits from the bottom. Reduce the heat to low, and stir in, a little at a time, the 1½ cups chicken broth while the mixture thickens.

4. Continue to stir over low heat for 5 more minutes, and then serve garnished with the scallions.

VARIATION 1 **CAULIFLOWER BREAKFAST RISOTTO:** Top the risotto with a fried or poached egg (see page 25). To fry an egg, crack one into a hot pan with ½ tablespoon grass-fed butter and cook until the white is no longer runny. Gently flip and cook to desired doneness (just a few seconds for over-easy, a minute or two for over-medium).

VARIATION 2 **CHICKEN-BACON CAULIFLOWER RISOTTO:** For some added protein, brown 1 or 2 diced chicken breasts in the pan with the mushrooms, garlic, and shallots. Continue with the recipe as written. Top with 2 tablespoons crumbled bacon.

PALEO PAIR: Serve with a side of Bacon Brussels Sprouts (page 178).

CAULIFLOWER FRITTERS

I had my first latke a few years ago at a friend's Hanukkah celebration, and I was completely blown away by how delicious they were. If you haven't had them before, they are savory little potato cakes usually served with sour cream and sliced scallions. This recipe is similar, but we skip the dairy and use cauliflower instead of potatoes. They make a nice side dish for steaks and chicken, but they'd also be a great appetizer the next time you're entertaining. **SERVES 4**

PREP TIME: 10 minutes
COOK TIME: 20 minutes

30

1 large head cauliflower, chopped into florets

1 or 2 garlic cloves, chopped

¼ cup almond flour

2 eggs

2 tablespoons grass-fed butter

2 tablespoons sliced scallions, for garnish

1. In a large pot of boiling water, quickly cook the cauliflower for 5 to 6 minutes, until barely fork-tender. Drain and allow to cool slightly. In a food processor or blender, chop the florets until they reach an almost mashed potato–like consistency.

2. Transfer to a bowl, and add the garlic, almond flour, and eggs. Stir until well incorporated.

3. In a large sauté pan over medium-high heat, melt the butter. Begin to cook the fritters: Spoon some of the cauliflower into your hand, create a patty about half the size of your palm, and carefully lower it into the butter. You should be able to cook 3 or 4 at a time without crowding the pan. Cook until browned on one side, about 3 minutes. Flip and cook the other side, about 3 minutes more.

4. Serve garnished with the scallions.

VARIATION 1 SWEET POTATO FRITTERS: Make this recipe with sweet potatoes. Dice 2 large sweet potatoes, and boil them for 10 to 15 minutes. Continue with the recipe as written. The frying time may be a few minutes longer, since sweet potatoes are more solid than cauliflower.

VARIATION 2 ORANGE-GINGER CARROT FRITTERS: Swap in carrots for the cauliflower (about 2 cups). The cook time should be about the same. Add ¼ teaspoon grated ginger and the zest of half an orange, and you'll have a sweet and spicy dish.

PREP TIP: Make the "batter" ahead of time, and then shape and fry them right before serving.

CAULIFLOWER TABBOULEH SALAD

This salad would be perfect for a light summer dinner—it's inspired by tabbouleh, which is a grain-based salad that usually has lemon, mint, parsley, cucumbers, and lots of lemon juice. As someone who eats a Paleo diet, I sometimes find myself missing out on trendy quinoa bowls at cute juice bars, so this one is for those afternoons when I want something light but still want to avoid rice and other grains. **SERVES 4**

PREP TIME: 20 minutes
COOK TIME: None

1 head cauliflower, cut into florets

2 to 3 cups your favorite salad mix (I like field greens with arugula)

½ red onion, diced

1 large cucumber, diced

10 ounces cherry tomatoes, halved

½ cup chopped fresh mint

¼ cup chopped fresh parsley

3 tablespoons extra-virgin olive oil

Juice of 2 or 3 lemons

Salt

Freshly ground black pepper

1. In a food processor or blender, "rice" the cauliflower—you want it to be pretty fine, but keep in mind that you're eating it raw and in a salad, so it needs to have some texture to it.

2. In a large serving bowl, combine the salad mix with the riced cauliflower, onion, cucumber, tomatoes, mint, and parsley. Toss, and drizzle the olive oil and lemon juice over it.

3. Season with salt and pepper, and toss again. Serve immediately.

VARIATION 1 **CAULIFLOWER RICE SALAD WITH BALSAMIC:** Skip the olive oil and lemon drizzle and serve with Balsamic Vinaigrette (page 89) for a sweeter version.

VARIATION 2 **CAULIFLOWER RICE SALAD WITH KALE, BACON, AND RANCH:** Use massaged kale (see page 119) instead of field greens. Skip the mint and parsley, and add 2 slices cooked crumbled bacon to the salad. Dress with Ranch Dressing (page 75).

PALEO PAIR: Serve alongside Chicken, Steak, or Shrimp Kebabs (page 98).

ROASTED CAULIFLOWER WITH TOMATOES AND BASIL

I think that roasting vegetables is probably the tastiest way to prepare any veggie, especially something kind of crunchy like cauliflower or broccoli. This recipe is a great side dish that you can customize with a bunch of different flavors, but you can't go wrong with tomatoes and lots of fresh basil. **SERVES 4**

PREP TIME: 10 minutes
COOK TIME: 40 minutes

1 large head cauliflower, cut into florets

1½ cups cherry tomatoes

2 to 3 tablespoons extra-virgin olive oil

1 tablespoon garlic powder

Salt

Freshly ground black pepper

¼ to ½ cup fresh basil, torn

2 tablespoons slivered almonds

1. Preheat the oven to 400°F.

2. On a large baking sheet, spread out the cauliflower florets and cherry tomatoes, and drizzle with the olive oil. Season with the garlic powder, salt, and pepper, and gently toss so the vegetables are well coated.

3. Bake for 20 to 30 minutes, checking halfway through the cooking time and moving them around with a spatula so all sides get browned. Leave them in for an additional 5 to 10 minutes if they aren't crisping up around the edges yet.

4. Transfer to a serving bowl, top with the basil and almonds, and serve.

VARIATION 1 **ROASTED CAULIFLOWER AND ASPARAGUS:** In spring, replace the tomatoes with 1 cup chopped asparagus and follow the recipe as written. Finish with a squeeze of lemon and fresh parsley instead of basil.

VARIATION 2 **ROASTED CAULIFLOWER WITH BROCCOLI AND TOMATOES:** For even more vegetables and variety, add 2 or 3 handfuls broccoli florets to the baking sheet. Add an extra teaspoon garlic powder to the mix, and bake according to the original recipe. Finish with a squeeze of lemon juice, if desired.

PALEO PAIR: This makes a great side to Shrimp Kebabs (page 98).

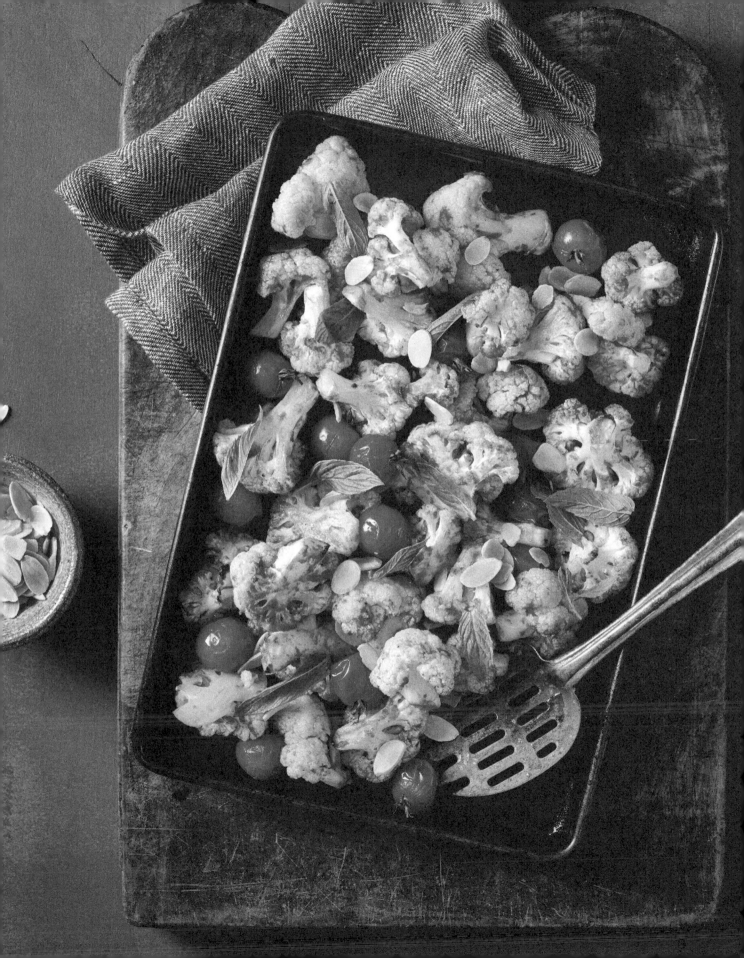

GENERAL TSO'S CAULIFLOWER

Whether you participate in Meatless Mondays or just love Asian food (I'm the latter and not so much the former), this spicy-sweet Chinese takeout–inspired cauliflower is going to knock your socks off. At the risk of repeating myself, I love Asian food more than most other things, so any time I can find a Paleo replacement for a cornstarch and sugar–laden craving, I'm game. **SERVES 4**

PREP TIME: 10 minutes
COOK TIME: 20 minutes

3 or 4 garlic cloves, minced

1 tablespoon minced fresh ginger

½ teaspoon red pepper flakes (more or less depending on heat preference)

1 tablespoon white vinegar

¼ cup extra-virgin olive oil

¼ cup sesame oil

¼ cup coconut aminos

1 tablespoon ghee

1 large head cauliflower, cut into florets with very short stems (to resemble bites of chicken)

¼ cup vegetable broth

Sesame seeds, for garnish

3 or 4 tablespoons sliced scallions, for garnish

1. In a large bowl, stir to combine the garlic, ginger, red pepper flakes, vinegar, olive oil, sesame oil, and coconut aminos.

2. In a large sauté pan over high heat, melt the ghee. Cook the cauliflower for 5 to 7 minutes, stirring frequently to prevent burning, until the cauliflower starts to brown.

3. Pour the sauce over the cauliflower, and cook for another 1 to 2 minutes. Reduce the heat to medium, and continue to stir. Bring the sauce to a simmer, and allow it to thicken. Pour in the vegetable broth, and deglaze the pan, stirring to scrape up the browned bits from the bottom.

4. Continue to cook until the cauliflower is fork-tender and the sauce is sticky and thick, about 10 minutes. Serve garnished with the sesame seeds and scallions.

VARIATION 1 **CASHEW CAULIFLOWER:** Top with a handful of cashews instead of sesame seeds before serving. These will add a nutty flavor and more of a bite to the dish.

VARIATION 2 **GENERAL TSO'S CAULIFLOWER SALAD:** Serve this cauliflower as a salad over a bed of cucumber noodles (see page 66) and ½ cup shredded cabbage.

PREP TIP: Make the sauce ahead of time (follow steps 1 and 3 without the cauliflower) and refrigerate so you can just reheat whenever you sauté the cauliflower.

WHOLE ROASTED CAULIFLOWER

Roasting a whole cauliflower is super easy and ends up looking somewhat impressive. It's a really beautiful dish, and you can make it with as few as three ingredients: a head of cauliflower, olive oil or melted butter or ghee, and some salt. We dress it up a little more for this recipe, but it's nice to know how to make it "plain" so you can customize it to your own tastes. **SERVES 4**

PREP TIME: 5 minutes
COOK TIME: 1 hour, 30 minutes

NF

1 large head cauliflower

¼ cup extra-virgin olive oil, melted butter, or ghee (be liberal with it!)

3 garlic cloves, minced

¼ cup chopped fresh thyme

Juice of ½ lemon

Salt

Freshly ground black pepper

1. Preheat the oven to 425°F.

2. Remove the leaves from the cauliflower, and carefully cut off the bottom stem so that the cauliflower can sit on a flat surface. In a small bowl, mix to combine the olive oil, garlic, thyme, and lemon juice.

3. Place the cauliflower on a baking sheet or in a cast iron skillet, and slowly pour the marinade over it. Rub it in as much as you can with your hands, and season generously with salt and pepper.

4. Roast for 1 to 1½ hours, or until the outside of the cauliflower is very roasted and brown.

5. Cut into wedges and serve.

VARIATION 1 **HONEY-MUSTARD WHOLE ROASTED CAULIFLOWER:** Before roasting the cauliflower as instructed, rub it with a mixture of 2 tablespoons grainy Dijon mustard, 2 tablespoons honey, and ¼ cup extra-virgin olive oil instead of the original marinade recipe. Season with salt and pepper.

VARIATION 2 **SPICY WHOLE ROASTED CAULIFLOWER:** Add 1 teaspoon chili powder and ¼ teaspoon ground cayenne pepper to the original marinade recipe. Skip the lemon juice, and roast according to the original recipe.

PALEO PAIR: Serve with Prosciutto-Wrapped Pork Tenderloin (page 73).

CAULIFLOWER

113

CURRY CAULIFLOWER BITES

Sometimes it seems that cauliflower gets a bad rep for being a little boring, but I think it's the opposite—because it has such a neutral flavor, it does well with a variety of spices. These roasted curry cauliflower bites work very well as a side dish or even a little appetizer before dinner. You could also serve them on top of a salad with some chicken if you want to make a light, flavorful lunch. **SERVES 4**

PREP TIME: 5 minutes
COOK TIME: 40 minutes

1 head cauliflower, cut into florets

3 tablespoons coconut oil, melted

1 tablespoon curry powder

1 teaspoon garlic powder

Salt

Freshly ground black pepper

1. Preheat the oven to 375°F.

2. In a large bowl, toss the cauliflower with the coconut oil, curry powder, and garlic powder, and season with salt and pepper.

3. Place the florets on a baking sheet, and roast for about 40 minutes, or until the cauliflower starts to get toasty and browned.

4. Serve immediately.

VARIATION 1 **BUFFALO CAULIFLOWER BITES:** Toss the cauliflower in homemade Buffalo Sauce (page 46), and roast according to the recipe.

VARIATION 2 **ROASTED CAULIFLOWER STEAKS:** Instead of cutting the cauliflower into florets, hold it on its side and slice it into two or three wider pieces, or "steaks." Season with a drizzle of olive oil, a pinch of salt, and a sprinkle of pepper, and roast at 400°F for 35 to 40 minutes.

PALEO PAIR: Serve alongside Curry Chicken (page 39) for an Indian-inspired dinner.

CAULIFLOWER SOUP

This is a great spring soup: It's pretty quick to make and super flavorful while still being neutral enough that you can add any variations you want. My friend Kristan once made a similar soup that had potatoes in it, which you can do if you aren't avoiding white potatoes—but the cauliflower is just lovely on its own. Here it is roasted with leeks, garlic, and onion to really bring out the flavors, and then it goes into a pot with chicken broth before being blended.

SERVES 4 TO 6

PREP TIME: 10 minutes
COOK TIME: 40 minutes

DF **NF**

4 large leeks, washed and thinly sliced (white and very light green parts only)

2 or 3 heads cauliflower, chopped into florets

4 or 5 garlic cloves, peeled

¼ cup extra-virgin olive oil

Salt

Freshly ground black pepper

3 cups chicken broth, divided

2 or 3 fresh thyme sprigs

1 or 2 tablespoons sliced scallions, for garnish

1. Preheat the oven to 400°F.

2. Season the leeks, cauliflower, and garlic with the olive oil, salt, and pepper. Divide the vegetables between 2 baking sheets, and roast for 20 to 30 minutes, or until slightly browned, rotating the pans halfway through the cooking time.

3. Remove from the oven, allow the vegetables to cool slightly, and then transfer them to a blender. Add 1½ cups of broth, and blend until smooth. Add the remaining 1½ cups of broth in increments and blend until your desired consistency is reached. If you have an immersion blender, you can put everything right into a large saucepan and blend on the stove.

4. Transfer the soup to a large saucepan, stir in the thyme, and simmer over low heat for 10 minutes. Add more chicken broth if the soup gets too thick.

5. Taste and add more salt and pepper if necessary, remove the thyme sprigs, and serve hot topped with the scallions.

VARIATION 1 **BROCCOLI-CAULIFLOWER SOUP:** Swap out the leeks for super healthy broccoli (about 2 cups broccoli and 2 cups cauliflower). Cook according to the recipe, and top with a couple tablespoons of cooked crumbled bacon.

VARIATION 2 **COCONUT CREAM–CAULIFLOWER SOUP:** To make this soup even creamier, add coconut cream to the pot and stir. To do this, refrigerate a can of coconut cream, and scoop out the solid part that rises to the top. (Discard the water that sits at the bottom or throw it into a smoothie.)

PALEO PAIR: Serve with a side of Golden Beet Salad (page 174).

CAULIFLOWER FRIED RICE

Fried rice is still one of my favorite "cheat" meals because it's relatively easy to make gluten-free, but I was so pleased when I finally perfected a Paleo, grain-free fried "rice." This one uses cauliflower instead of rice, and coconut aminos instead of soy sauce, but the most important ingredient is the same, and that's butter, which helps you get those delicious toasty bites of rice, or in our case, cauliflower. **SERVES 4**

PREP TIME: 5 minutes
COOK TIME: 15 minutes

1 head cauliflower, cut into florets

1½ tablespoons sesame oil

1 to 2 tablespoons grass-fed butter

1 garlic clove, minced

¼ teaspoon minced fresh ginger

¼ cup diced carrots

¼ cup green peas (thawed if frozen)

¼ teaspoon red pepper flakes

2 tablespoons coconut aminos

1 egg

1 to 2 tablespoons sliced scallions, for garnish

Freshly ground black pepper

1. In a food processor or blender, roughly chop the cauliflower florets. You want it to be the consistency of regular rice.

2. In a large skillet over medium heat, heat the sesame oil. Spread the riced cauliflower out in a single layer, and let it cook for about 2 minutes, and then stir it up and repeat several times, for a total of 5 to 7 minutes.

3. Add the butter, garlic, and ginger, and stir until well incorporated. Add the carrots, peas, red pepper flakes, and coconut aminos, and continue to stir.

4. Make an opening in the center of the pan by moving everything to the edges. Crack the egg over the pan and scramble it quickly. Incorporate the scrambled egg into the fried rice.

5. Continue to cook until the cauliflower starts getting crispy (feel free to add another half tablespoon or so of butter if you wish), another 5 to 7 minutes.

6. Stir in the scallions, season with pepper, and serve.

VARIATION 1 **PLAIN CAULIFLOWER RICE:** Sauté the riced cauliflower over medium heat in 1 to 2 tablespoons olive oil, and add salt and pepper to taste.

VARIATION 2 **DAIKON FRIED RICE:** Use daikon root instead of cauliflower—chop it in the food processor the same way. Daikon has a slightly spicy radish flavor, so I like to use it in smaller amounts than the cauliflower. Or you could mix it up and use a bit of both.

PALEO PAIR: Serve with Shrimp Stir-Fry (page 96) or Ground Pork Stir-Fry (page 67).

PANTRY BASIC: NOT-SPINACH ARTICHOKE DIP

My mom and I make this dip all the time—it was inspired by a recipe my friend Melissa used to make with hearts of palm, which was, in turn, inspired by a big ol' charcuterie snack platter my mom made for us once, which just happened to include big pieces of hearts of palm. She thought the texture was similar to string cheese. I added artichoke hearts and jalapeño to her original recipe to make a Paleo spin on cheesy spinach-artichoke dip. **MAKES 3 TO 4 CUPS**

PREP TIME: 5 minutes
COOK TIME: None

`30` `NF` `V`

1 (14-ounce) can hearts of palm

1 (14-ounce) can artichoke hearts

¼ fresh jalapeño pepper

Juice of ½ lemon

3 garlic cloves

3 tablespoons extra-virgin olive oil

1. Drain the hearts of palm and artichoke hearts, and transfer them to a food processor or blender. Add the jalapeño, lemon juice, and garlic, and blend until roughly chopped. Turn the food processor back on, and keep it running while you drizzle the olive oil in.

2. Scoop the dip out and serve with carrots, celery, and/or Sweet Potato Chips (page 219).

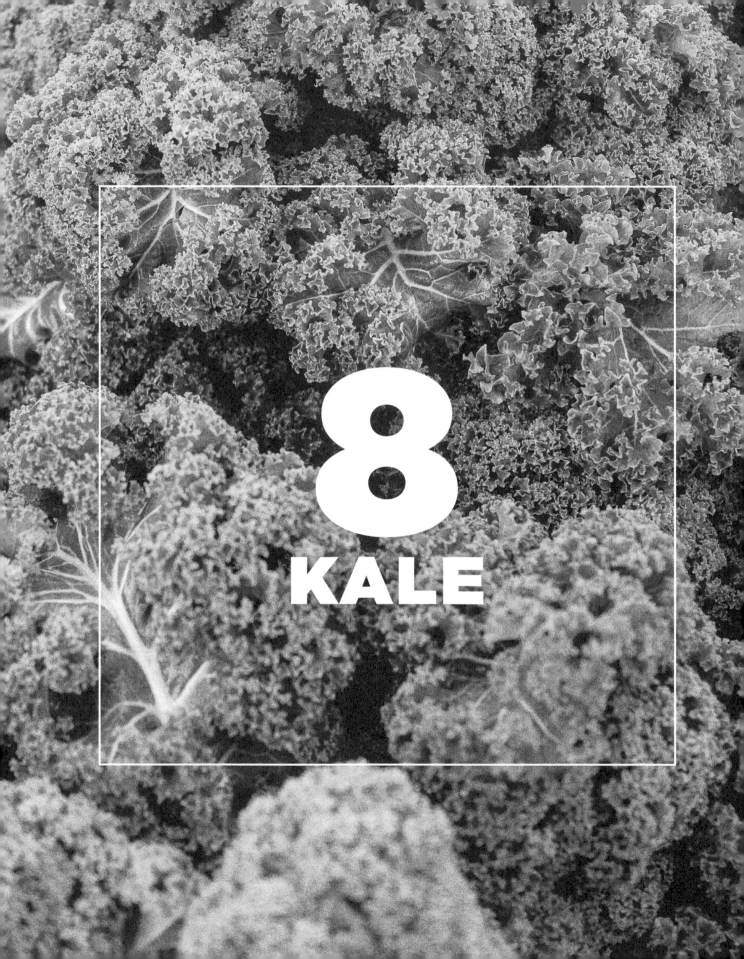

8
KALE

Kale has got to be the trendiest vegetable right now, which I find pretty funny. I love reading about food trends and seeing what's popular and what isn't anymore, especially when it's something as simple as a vegetable. Doughnuts, cronuts, and macarons I get, but when it comes to kale and Brussels sprouts, you'd think some things just never go out of style.

An important note that I want to be sure everyone knows: Kale can be super delicious when served raw in a salad, but you really have to massage it first. I like to pour a little olive oil on it and use my hands to work it in (then you can add whatever other dressing you're planning to use). Do this for at least 4 to 5 minutes, or until the leaves are all coated with oil and start to turn dark green. This makes them less tough and a lot easier to eat raw.

In this chapter I've included recipes for salads, cooked kale, kale chips, and even a smoothie. Sometimes I avoid buying a big bag of the greens because I worry that I won't get through it before they start to wilt, but with the ten recipes below, you can buy in bulk with complete peace of mind.

GREEN SMOOTHIES

I love having a smoothie for breakfast or a snack when it's hot outside—especially if I'm starting to get sick of scrambled eggs, which I make for breakfast approximately every single morning. My favorite way to make a smoothie is with a really huge handful of greens. A big serving of vegetables makes me feel like I'm starting my day on the right foot. **SERVES 2**

PREP TIME: 5 minutes
COOK TIME: None

1 to 2 cups chopped kale leaves

½ cup diced pineapple

1 tablespoon (about a 1-inch chunk) fresh ginger, peeled

¼ cup freshly squeezed orange juice

1 handful ice

1. In a blender, blend the kale, pineapple, and ginger until they start to combine.

2. Add the orange juice and ice, and blend until smooth. If it's too thick, add another splash of juice and blend again.

3. Pour into 2 glasses and serve.

VARIATION 1 **GREEN SMOOTHIES WITH SPINACH:** Swap the kale for well-washed and drained spinach if you like it more or happen to have it in your refrigerator.

VARIATION 2 **STRAWBERRY-BANANA GREEN SMOOTHIES:** Blend 1 ripe banana, ¾ cup strawberries, and 1 to 2 cups chopped kale with ¼ cup almond or coconut milk and a handful of ice.

PREP TIP: Buy frozen fruit instead of fresh (or chop your own fruit and then freeze it) so you can skip the ice and have a more concentrated smoothie.

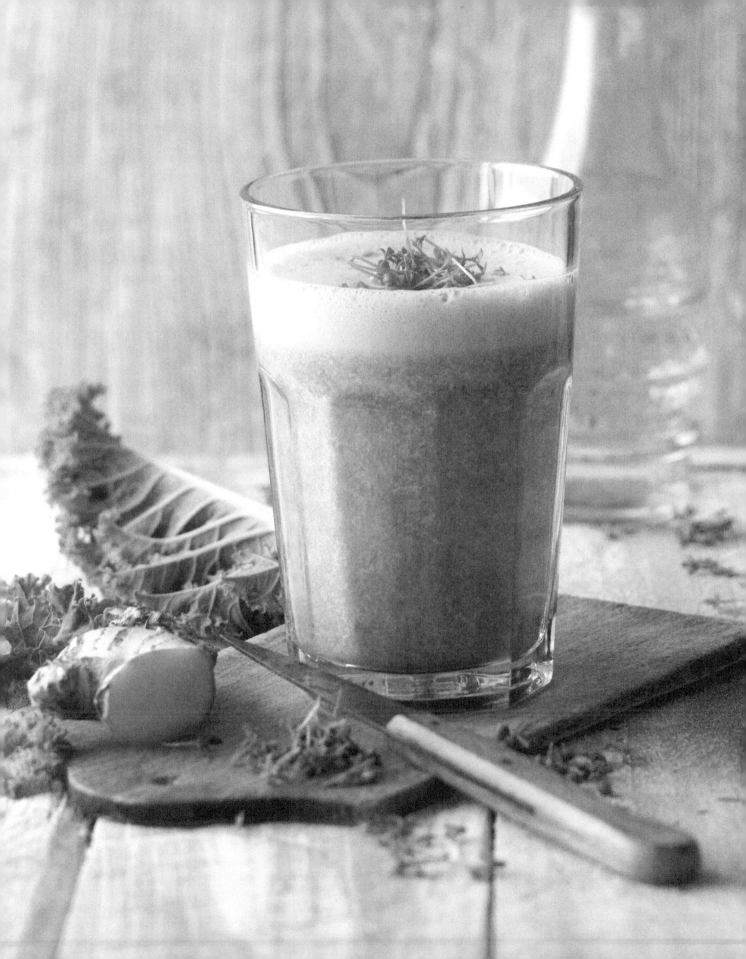

KALE CHIPS

Kale chips are really easy to make, and they're perfect for when you buy a huge bag of kale at the store and then forget about it until it's about to wilt and get soggy, so you have to use all of it at once (or is that just me?). You can make these spicy or plain and add all kinds of different flavors and spices to them, so spend some time experimenting to discover your perfect kale chip. **SERVES 4**

PREP TIME: 5 minutes
COOK TIME: 15 minutes

1 large head kale, stemmed

2 tablespoons extra-virgin olive oil

Salt

Freshly ground black pepper

1. Preheat the oven to 350°F.

2. Wash and dry the kale before tearing or cutting it into bite-size pieces. Lay them out on a baking sheet, and sprinkle with the olive oil. Season with salt and pepper. Mix everything up with your hands to make sure all the leaves are coated with olive oil.

3. Bake until crispy, 12 to 15 minutes, keeping an eye on them so they don't burn.

4. Serve immediately.

VARIATION 1 **SPICY KALE CHIPS:** Season the kale with ¼ teaspoon ground cayenne pepper or red pepper flakes.

VARIATION 2 **SALT AND VINEGAR KALE CHIPS:** Season the kale chips with oil, salt, and pepper as directed in step 2, but add 2 or 3 teaspoons of white vinegar as well.

PREP TIP: Kale chips don't do well as leftovers, so make them an even faster recipe by cutting the stems out and tearing your kale ahead of time. If you want, you can then marinate them in olive oil, so they'll be extra flavorful and crunchy.

SIMPLE SAUTÉED KALE

This is the most basic of kale recipes, and yet one of my favorites. I like to use it as a base for all sorts of proteins—I just plate it and put chicken or shrimp or whatever else I happen to be making that night right on top. You can customize it however you like to capture your favorite flavors, but I always think it should start, like most things, with onion, garlic, and some butter or olive oil. **SERVES 4**

PREP TIME: 5 minutes
COOK TIME: 20 minutes

30 **NF**

1 tablespoon grass-fed butter or extra-virgin olive oil

¼ to ½ onion, diced

2 garlic cloves, minced

10 ounces kale, stemmed and chopped

Salt

Freshly ground black pepper

1. In a large skillet over medium heat, melt the butter. Sauté the onion until slightly translucent, about 5 minutes. Add the garlic, giving it a stir, and cook for another 1 to 2 minutes.

2. Add the kale to the pan a couple of handfuls at a time, stirring gently as the leaves wilt. Cook the kale for about 10 minutes, until it is all wilted.

3. Season with salt and pepper and serve.

VARIATION 1 **SAUTÉED ASIAN KALE:** Use sesame oil instead of butter or olive oil. Season with 1 to 2 teaspoons chili paste, and garnish with 1 tablespoon sesame seeds.

VARIATION 2 **CURRIED KALE:** Sauté the onion, garlic, and kale according to the original recipe, and then add 2 teaspoons curry powder and 1 tablespoon canned coconut milk.

PALEO PAIR: Serve sautéed kale with or on Burger Bowls (page 51).

SOUTHERN-STYLE KALE GREENS

Living in the South means there are some seriously good collard greens to be had. They're slow-cooked in bacon and broth and delicious as a side with BBQ or chicken. I love them but don't always find collards as easily as I do kale, and as I often buy a big bag of kale at the grocery store, I decided to make a kale version of the classic Southern dish. **SERVES 4**

PREP TIME: 10 minutes
COOK TIME: 30 minutes

3 slices bacon

1 onion, sliced

3 garlic cloves, minced

10 ounces chopped kale

1 tablespoon honey

2 teaspoons apple cider vinegar

½ cup chicken broth

Salt

Freshly ground black pepper

1. In a medium saucepan over medium-high heat, fry the bacon until crispy, about 5 minutes. Set aside. In the same pan, sauté the onion and garlic together for about 5 minutes, or until the onion becomes slightly translucent.

2. Add the kale to the pan, and stir well so that it begins to wilt evenly, about 5 minutes. Add the honey, and continue to stir. Pour in the apple cider vinegar.

3. Pour in the broth, and bring to a simmer. Reduce the heat to low, and cook for about 10 minutes, or until the kale is completely tender. Season with salt and pepper.

4. Use tongs or a slotted spoon to serve.

VARIATION 1 **COLLARD GREENS:** For even more fiber, make this recipe with 10 ounces collard greens instead of kale (the cook time should be about the same).

VARIATION 2 **SOUTHERN-STYLE GREENS WITH PANCETTA:** Make these greens (either kale or collards) with pancetta instead of bacon. Although bacon and pancetta are very similar, pancetta is unsmoked, so if you prefer less of a smoky taste to your pork, try that instead.

PALEO PAIR: Serve these with the Baby Back Ribs (page 70).

RAW ZUCCHINI NOODLE-PESTO SALAD

I'm not a big fan of the whole hide-the-veggies-so-kids-don't-know-they're-eating-it thing, but then again, I don't have kids, so my opinion is not really important. However, if you can add vegetables to something without altering the taste that much, I'm all in. This pesto is similar to the one you'll find on page 175, except it's loaded with kale, so you get an extra serving of greens every time you use it. It's a pretty good deal, if you ask me. **SERVES 4**

PREP TIME: 15 minutes
COOK TIME: None

2 cups stemmed and roughly chopped kale leaves

1 cup fresh basil leaves

¼ cup pine nuts

½ cup extra-virgin olive oil

Salt

Freshly ground black pepper

1 cup raw zucchini noodles (see page 125)

1. In a food processor or blender, roughly chop the kale, basil, and pine nuts, stopping occasionally to push all the leaves down from the sides with a spatula. Turn the food processor back on, and slowly drizzle in the olive oil. Season with salt and pepper.

2. In a serving bowl, spoon the kale pesto over the zucchini noodles. Toss well and serve.

VARIATION 1 **RAW ZUCCHINI NOODLE–PESTO SALAD WITH CHICKEN:** Top the main recipe with 4 to 6 ounces diced chicken breast. (Salmon would also be delicious if you feel like fish instead.)

VARIATION 2 **KALE PESTO WITH WALNUTS:** Replace the pine nuts with walnuts for a less expensive pesto. Top your dish with extra walnuts.

PREP TIP: Pesto freezes really well, so make a big batch and freeze it in small containers or even in an ice cube tray.

KALE CHICKEN SALAD

This recipe is inspired by a "sandwich" I once had at a Mediterranean restaurant in Charlotte. I ordered it without the bread because it sounded like it would be a really nice piece of lemon-oregano chicken, but what came out was a huge pile of chicken salad with lots of greens mixed in. I was so pleasantly surprised and delighted because that's something I normally wouldn't have ordered, and now I make it for myself at home. **SERVES 4**

PREP TIME: 10 minutes, plus 15 minutes to marinate
COOK TIME: None

30 **DF** **NF**

2 (12.5-ounce) cans chicken

1 heaping cup shredded kale

½ cucumber, diced

¼ cup sliced Kalamata olives

¼ cup chopped tomato

¼ cup chopped fresh mint leaves

2 tablespoons Homemade Mayo (page 47)

2 teaspoons dried oregano

Juice of 2 lemons

Salt

Freshly ground black pepper

In a large bowl, stir well to combine the chicken, kale, cucumber, olives, tomato, mint, Homemade Mayo, oregano, and lemon juice. Season with salt and pepper, and allow the salad to marinate in the refrigerator for 10 to 15 minutes before serving.

VARIATION 1 **KALE CHICKEN SALAD OVER GREENS:** Although this salad is just great on its own, you can double your veggies and have it for lunch over a bed of field greens.

VARIATION 2 **KALE SALMON SALAD:** Use 18 ounces canned (or fresh) salmon instead of chicken to boost your omega-3 levels.

PREP TIP: If you don't have canned chicken, just use 1 pound boneless skinless chicken breasts. Gently poach them in water by bringing them to a boil and then reducing to a simmer for about 15 minutes, and then shred them once they've cooled.

KALE SALAD WITH PECANS AND APPLES

Kale seems like it's too tough to serve raw, but when it's dressed and massaged a bit (even just with wooden spoons while tossing with dressing), it becomes really tender and stands up well to nuts, fruit, and other salad additions that at other times can seem too much. This one is loaded with pecans, bacon, and apple and dressed with a refreshingly tangy apple cider vinaigrette. **SERVES 6 TO 8**

PREP TIME: 10 minutes
COOK TIME: 10 minutes

5 to 6 cups stemmed, chopped kale leaves

2 tablespoons extra-virgin olive oil, plus ½ tablespoon for massaging

1 tablespoon coconut oil

1 cup pecans

6 slices bacon

2 tablespoons honey

1 tablespoon apple cider vinegar

1 tablespoon Dijon mustard

¼ teaspoon red pepper flakes

Freshly ground black pepper

1 green apple, skinned and sliced

1. In a large bowl, drizzle the kale with ½ tablespoon of olive oil. Massage the leaves really well with your hands for a few minutes to tenderize the leaves.

2. In a large skillet over medium-low heat, melt the coconut oil. Toast the pecans until they just start to brown, about 5 minutes, watching them carefully so they don't burn. Set aside.

3. In a separate large skillet over medium-high heat, cook the bacon until crispy, about 5 minutes. Set the bacon aside, and transfer the bacon grease to a small bowl for the salad dressing. Combine it with the honey, apple cider vinegar, Dijon mustard, and red pepper flakes. Season with pepper, and drizzle the remaining 2 tablespoons of olive oil into the bowl while whisking the dressing.

4. Assemble the salad by putting the kale in a large serving bowl and topping with the toasted pecans and sliced apples. Toss with the dressing, and serve.

VARIATION 1 CRANBERRY-KALE SALAD: Swap the apples for 1 cup dried cranberries for a tarter taste.

VARIATION 2 ARUGULA SALAD: Swap in arugula for the kale—I love arugula because it has a bright, almost bitter flavor to it. You don't need to massage the arugula, as it is already tender.

PALEO PAIR: Serve this salad with Prosciutto-Wrapped Pork Tenderloin (page 73).

KALE SALAD WITH ONION AND AVOCADO

I had a salad similar to this one at a place called Oddfellows in Seattle—I had just landed; my friend Kristan picked me up, and we went right to lunch. I was starving and tired from the cross-country trip but so excited to be there that I downed a cortado followed by a glass of rosé. I ordered a kale salad that was mixed with romaine and topped with onion and avocado. It was such a simple meal, but one that I'll remember for a long time. **SERVES 2**

PREP TIME: 10 minutes
COOK TIME: None

FOR THE SALAD

5 ounces kale, stemmed and chopped

5 ounces romaine lettuce, chopped

¼ red onion, thinly sliced

1 avocado, quartered and thinly sliced

FOR THE DRESSING

2 tablespoons balsamic vinegar

1½ teaspoons Dijon mustard

1 tablespoon honey

4 tablespoons extra-virgin olive oil

Salt

Freshly ground black pepper

TO MAKE THE SALAD

In a large bowl, toss to combine the kale and romaine. Top with the red onion and avocado.

TO MAKE THE DRESSING

In a small bowl, whisk together the balsamic vinegar, Dijon mustard, and honey. While whisking, drizzle in the olive oil. Season with salt and pepper. Pour the dressing over the salad and toss well, making sure all the kale has been coated, and serve.

VARIATION 1 **CHICKEN-KALE SALAD WITH ONION AND AVOCADO:** Add 6 to 8 ounces diced or shredded cooked chicken breast to this salad to make it more of a main dish. (You might want to add another teaspoon or two of dressing.)

VARIATION 2 **SPINACH-KALE SALAD WITH ONION AND SALMON:** Add a couple of handfuls of well-washed and drained spinach leaves to the salad, and top with 6 to 8 ounces cooked salmon. (You don't need to massage the already-tender spinach.)

PREP TIP: Make the salad ahead of time and dress right before serving.

TURKEY-BACON-AVOCADO KALE WRAPS

Paleo lunches are usually just leftovers or salads, so there are times when I definitely miss wraps and sandwiches. Usually I'll make lettuce wraps, and those are good, but they aren't really as flexible as a traditional tortilla. I prefer to use a cabbage, collard, or kale leaf because they're sturdier and just a bit more wrap-like. **SERVES 1**

PREP TIME: 5 minutes
COOK TIME: None

1 large kale leaf, most of the stem removed

4 slices cooked turkey

Homemade Mayo (page 47) or Ranch Dressing (page 75), for spreading

¼ avocado, sliced

1 slice cooked bacon

1 slice tomato, halved (optional)

Place the kale leaf on a cutting board. Layer the turkey onto the leaf, and spread a bit of Mayo or Ranch Dressing over it. Add the avocado, bacon, and tomato (if using) on top of the turkey, roll it up, and serve.

VARIATION 1 **BUFFALO CHICKEN–KALE WRAP:** Cut a chicken breast into long slices, and toss with Buffalo Sauce (page 46). Wrap in a kale leaf, and serve with Ranch Dressing (page 75).

VARIATION 2 **CHICKEN SALAD WRAP:** Wrap Chicken Salad (page 38) in a kale leaf.

PREP TIP: Make these the night before so they're ready for work or school lunches.

SAUSAGE AND KALE SOUP

This sausage and kale soup reminds me a lot of Italian Wedding Soup, which I loved as a kid. Italian Wedding Soup consists of flavorful broth, small meatballs, and lots of greens. This soup is similar but comes together a little faster by using sausage instead of homemade meatballs. If you have them cooked already, you can just slice them up, or cook them quickly while you make your broth. This soup is perfect for a rainy lunch or dinner. **SERVES 4**

PREP TIME: 10 minutes
COOK TIME: 20 minutes

1 tablespoon extra-virgin olive oil

1 onion, diced

2 garlic cloves, minced

¼ to ½ teaspoon red pepper flakes

Salt

Freshly ground black pepper

10 to 12 ounces kale, stemmed and chopped

4 to 5 cups chicken broth

10 to 12 ounces cooked sausage, cut into slices

1. In a large saucepan over medium heat, heat the olive oil. Sauté the onion until slightly translucent, about 5 minutes. Add the garlic and red pepper flakes, season with salt and pepper, and give it a stir.

2. Add the kale, and sauté for another 2 minutes. Pour in the chicken broth, and bring to a simmer. Add the sausage, reduce the heat to low, and continue to stir periodically while cooking for an additional 10 to 15 minutes.

3. Serve hot.

VARIATION 1 **SAUSAGE AND KALE SWEET POTATO SOUP:** Dice 1 large sweet potato, and sauté it with the onion and garlic. Continue with the rest of the recipe as written.

VARIATION 2 **CHICKEN AND KALE SOUP:** For a lighter meal, substitute the sausage with either cooked chicken sausage or shredded chicken breast (10 to 12 ounces).

PREP TIP: Make a double batch of this soup, and freeze it in smaller portions. I like to defrost it in a saucepan over low heat and serve it immediately.

PANTRY BASIC: BBQ SAUCE

BBQ sauce is such a delicious condiment, but it's usually full of sugar, so my brother (who isn't Paleo but just loves me a lot and enjoys experimenting in the kitchen) came up with a pretty awesome Paleo-friendly BBQ sauce for us. I think the magic ingredient is pineapple juice, which lends sweetness to the sauce without the need for any added sugar. **MAKES ABOUT 2 CUPS**

PREP TIME: 5 minutes
COOK TIME: 1 hour

DF **NF**

1 cup apple cider vinegar

1 cup white vinegar

Zest and juice of ½ lemon

¼ cup honey

1 teaspoon garlic powder

1 teaspoon onion powder

1 teaspoon ground paprika

½ teaspoon freshly ground black pepper

½ teaspoon ground cayenne pepper (or less if you don't want it super spicy)

½ teaspoon red pepper flakes

1 heaping teaspoon tomato paste

¾ cup pineapple juice

1. In a medium saucepan over medium heat, stir together the apple cider vinegar, white vinegar, lemon zest and juice, honey, garlic powder, onion powder, paprika, black pepper, cayenne pepper, red pepper flakes, tomato paste, and pineapple juice until smooth. Bring to a simmer.

2. Reduce the heat to low and cook, stirring occasionally, for at least 30 minutes, but closer to 1 hour if you have time.

3. Remove from the heat, cool, and store in a mason jar or other container with a tightly fitting lid.

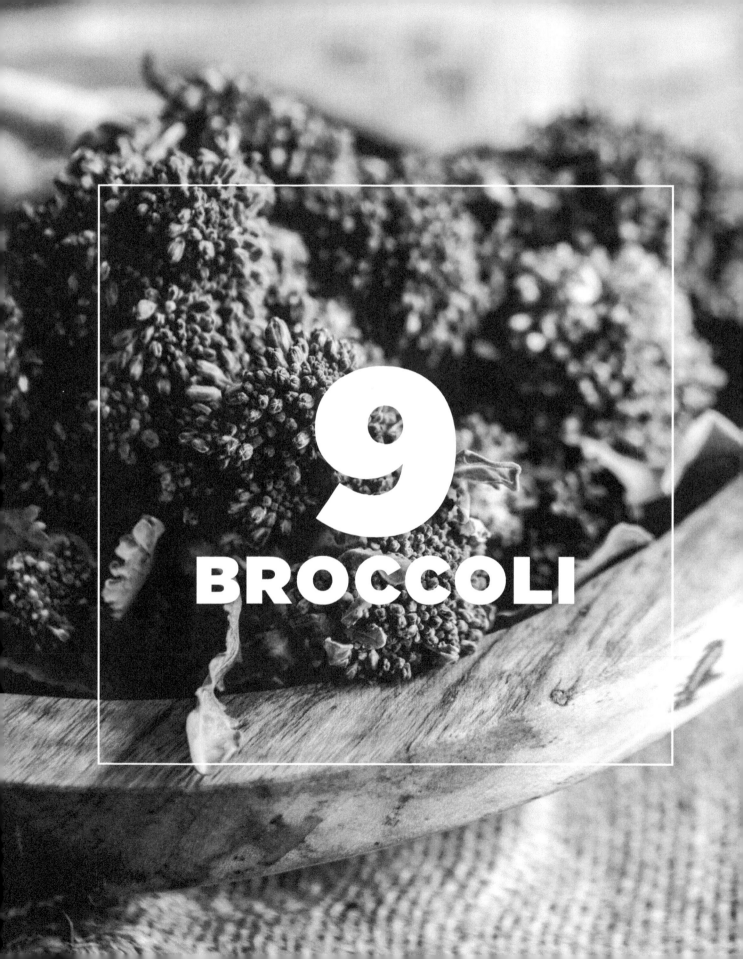

9
BROCCOLI

For me, broccoli is a nostalgic veggie—I have vivid memories of eating it steamed with a little butter as a kid (and I love the grown-up version with homemade hollandaise sauce on page 142). The Broccoli Salad recipe (page 137) with mayo, cranberries, and almonds is also one that I grew up eating, and it's still a favorite.

Broccoli goes far beyond the steamer basket, adapting to many cooking techniques and flavor combinations. You'll never go wrong roasting it with a little lemon juice—so simple and so delicious! The Broccoli Wraps (page 141) are my new favorite way to prep for lunch—I make them on Sunday night and stuff them with turkey, avocado, and homemade mayo throughout the week. I've found that eating Paleo is never hard when you've done the prep work and have all your meals planned, especially lunch.

BROCCOLI SLAW

This broccoli slaw is a great recipe for your next cookout—it's a little sweet and a little tangy, and it goes really well as a side to almost anything. You can easily make it ahead of time; in fact, it's even better if you do—like most slaws, the longer it all has to marinate together, the better the flavors will be.

SERVES 4 TO 6

PREP TIME: 10 minutes, plus 1 hour to marinate
COOK TIME: 5 minutes

DF

10 ounces broccoli coleslaw mix

5 ounces red cabbage, chopped

2 tablespoons apple cider vinegar

1 tablespoon honey

1 tablespoon Dijon mustard

¼ cup extra-virgin olive oil

½ cup sliced almonds

1 to 2 tablespoons sliced scallions, for garnish

1. In a large bowl, toss to combine the broccoli coleslaw mix with the red cabbage.

2. In a small bowl, whisk together the apple cider vinegar, honey, and Dijon mustard. While whisking, drizzle in the olive oil. Pour the dressing over the slaw, and mix well. Refrigerate for at least an hour.

3. In a dry pan over medium-low heat, toast the sliced almonds, watching carefully so they don't burn. Remove from the heat as soon as they begin to brown and smell fragrant, about 5 minutes.

4. Top the salad with the toasted almonds and scallions before serving.

VARIATION 1 **BROCCOLI SLAW WITH DRIED CRANBERRIES:** Add ½ cup dried cranberries to the slaw.

VARIATION 2 **BROCCOLI SLAW WITH PANCETTA:** Add ¼ cup diced, cooked pancetta (if it's raw, you can quickly pan-fry it before throwing it in).

PREP TIP: Make this slaw the night before so it has plenty of time to soak up all the flavors, and you'll have one less thing to do before serving.

ROASTED BROCCOLI WITH LEMON

This is by far my favorite way to cook broccoli—roasting it makes it delightfully crispy and flavorful. I'm a big fan of garlic and lemon together, especially when it comes to roasted green veggies (I like making Brussels sprouts and green beans the same way). Whether you're serving fish, chicken, or beef, roasted broccoli with lemon and garlic will always be a hit. **SERVES 4**

PREP TIME: 5 minutes
COOK TIME: 20 minutes

1 large head broccoli, cut into florets

4 tablespoons extra-virgin olive oil

Garlic powder, for seasoning

Salt

Freshly ground black pepper

Juice of 1 lemon

1. Preheat the oven to 450°F.

2. On a large baking sheet, drizzle the broccoli florets with the olive oil. Season generously with garlic powder, salt, and pepper. Use your hands to mix, making sure the broccoli florets are thoroughly coated.

3. Bake for 15 to 20 minutes, mixing with a spatula halfway through the cooking time.

4. Pour the lemon juice over the roasted broccoli, toss, and serve.

VARIATION 1 **ROASTED BROCCOLI WITH LEMON AND TAHINI:** Mix ½ cup tahini with the lemon juice, and season with salt and pepper. Toss the broccoli in the sauce, or use it as a dip.

VARIATION 2 **SPICY ROASTED BROCCOLI:** Add ¼ teaspoon red pepper flakes to the seasoning before roasting.

PALEO PAIR: Serve as a side with Sea Bass Topped with Crab (page 88).

BROCCOLI SOUP

My husband doesn't like soup all that much so I don't often make it at home, but this broccoli soup is perfect for whipping up anytime you're in the mood. It's kind of a Paleo version of cream of broccoli: just some onions, garlic, lots of broccoli, chicken broth, and a little coconut milk for creaminess.

SERVES 4 TO 6

PREP TIME: 10 minutes
COOK TIME: 25 minutes

NF

2 tablespoons grass-fed butter

1 small onion, diced

2 garlic cloves, minced

3 to 4 cups chicken broth

1 large head broccoli (and most of the stem), cut into florets

1 (13.5-ounce) can full-fat coconut milk

Salt

Freshly ground black pepper

1. In a large saucepan over medium heat, melt the butter. Sauté the onion until slightly translucent, about 5 minutes. Add the garlic, and stir, cooking for an additional 2 to 3 minutes. Pour the chicken broth into the pan, and bring to a boil. Add the broccoli, and stir.

2. Reduce the heat to a simmer, and cook for 10 to 15 minutes, or until the broccoli has softened.

3. Add the coconut milk, season with salt and pepper, and either transfer to a blender or use an immersion blender to blend the soup until it is smooth.

4. Serve hot.

VARIATION 1 **BROCCOLI-LEEK SOUP:** Add 1 large sliced leek (only the white and very light green parts) to the pan with the garlic if you'd like a springier version of this soup. Garnish with sliced scallions.

VARIATION 2 **BACON-BROCCOLI SOUP:** Cook 3 or 4 slices of chopped bacon in the saucepan, set aside, and cook the onion and garlic in the bacon grease. Continue with the recipe as written, and top the finished soup with the crumbled bacon.

PALEO PAIR: This soup is great as a light lunch with lots of field greens topped with Beet and Citrus Salad (page 165).

BROCCOLI SALAD

I really enjoy rediscovering recipes that I grew up with and realizing that they're Paleo. My mom used to make this salad whenever we'd have people over for a casual summer party, and even though it wasn't my favorite as a kid, it's one of my favorites now. There's just something about the combination of broccoli and mayo that I love—I actually dip steamed broccoli in mayo all the time! The next time you're making mayonnaise, prepare a double batch, and you'll be ready to whip this salad up in no time. **SERVES 4**

PREP TIME: 10 minutes, plus 20 minutes to rest
COOK TIME: None

30 **DF**

FOR THE DRESSING
½ cup Homemade Mayo (page 47)

¼ red onion, finely diced

1 tablespoon red wine vinegar

2 teaspoons honey

Pinch salt

Pinch freshly ground black pepper

FOR THE SALAD
1 large head broccoli, cut into bite-size pieces

½ cup dried cranberries

½ cup toasted almonds (see page 78)

TO MAKE THE DRESSING

In a small bowl, stir well to combine the Homemade Mayo, red onion, vinegar, honey, salt, and pepper. Set aside.

TO MAKE THE SALAD

1. In a large bowl, toss the broccoli and cranberries with the dressing. Top with the toasted almonds.

2. If possible, wait about 20 minutes before serving to allow the dressing to fully combine with the broccoli.

VARIATION 1 **BROCCOLI SALAD WITH RAISINS:** Swap the cranberries for raisins if you're looking for a less tart version.

VARIATION 2 **BACON-BROCCOLI SALAD:** Mix 3 or 4 cooked and crumbled slices bacon into the dressing before tossing.

PALEO PAIR: Serve as a side (or a topping) with Burger Bowls (page 51).

BROCCOLI-ARUGULA SALAD WITH BACON

I almost always have the ingredients for this simple salad in my refrigerator, but I often forget to throw them all together. Broccoli and cucumber are both such "snacky" vegetables in my mind—I never do much more with them than cut them up and munch on them with a side of Ranch Dressing (page 75), but they are so good for adding texture and flavor to salads. Add a little red onion and some bacon, and you've got lunch. **SERVES 4**

PREP TIME: 10 minutes
COOK TIME: None

2 cups arugula, washed and well drained

½ cup broccoli florets

½ cucumber, quartered and sliced

¼ red onion, thinly sliced

3 to 4 tablespoons apple cider vinaigrette (see page 179)

2 or 3 slices cooked bacon, cut widthwise into strips

In a large bowl, toss to combine the arugula, broccoli, cucumber, and red onion with the vinaigrette. Top with the bacon strips, and serve.

VARIATION 1 **BROCCOLI-SPINACH SALAD WITH PECANS AND APPLES:** Add ¼ cup toasted pecans and half a diced green apple to the salad.

VARIATION 2 **BROCCOLI-SPINACH SALAD WITH BACON:** Swap out the arugula for spinach if you're in the mood for a less peppery salad. (You can also skip the bacon if you want only veggies.)

PALEO PAIR: Serve with Baby Back Ribs (page 70).

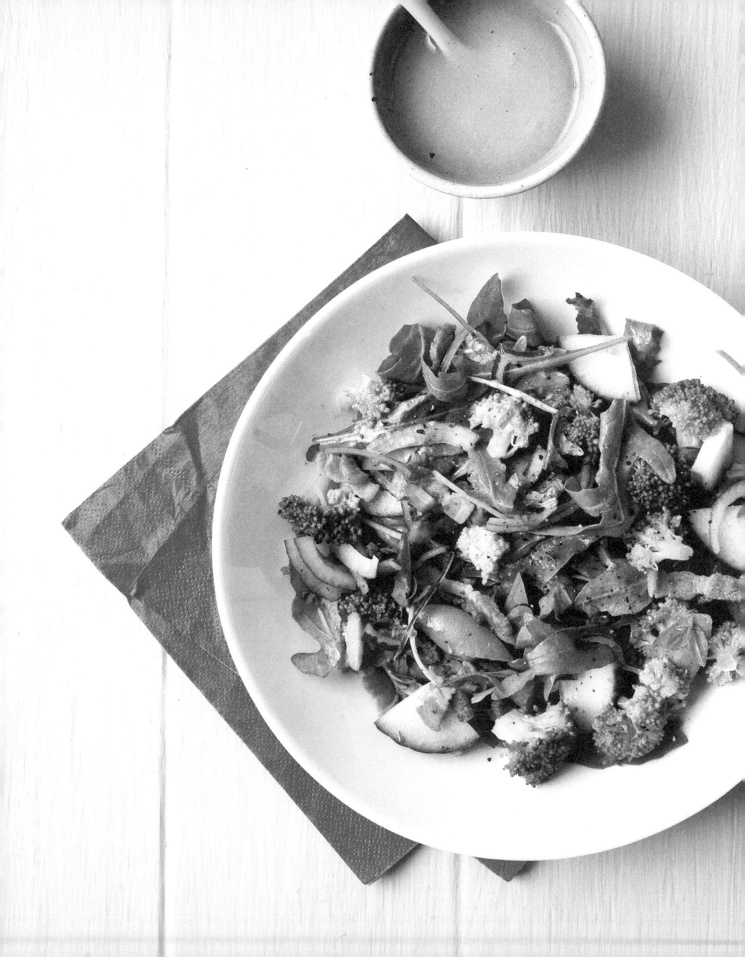

CRUSTLESS BROCCOLI TORTE

This crustless broccoli torte is kind of like a casserole, except that the eggs aren't the main ingredient the way they are in a more traditional breakfast casserole. The star of this show is broccoli, and here it is mixed with artichoke hearts and some almond flour. It makes a great breakfast but also a delicious appetizer or veggie side dish to almost any dinner you can think of. **SERVES 4**

PREP TIME: 10 minutes
COOK TIME: 50 minutes

1 large head broccoli, cut into florets

1 (14-ounce) can artichoke hearts, drained and chopped

2 eggs

½ red onion, diced

¼ cup almond milk

2 tablespoons almond flour

1 teaspoon garlic powder

Salt

Freshly ground black pepper

1 tablespoon grass-fed butter

1. Preheat the oven to 350°F.

2. In a medium pot over medium-high heat, lightly boil the broccoli for 2 to 3 minutes, or until almost fork-tender. Drain well, transfer to a food processor or blender, and pulse until roughly chopped.

3. Transfer to a large bowl, and add the artichoke hearts, eggs, onion, almond milk, almond flour, and garlic powder. Season with salt and pepper, and stir well.

4. Grease an 8-inch round baking pan with the butter, and transfer the mixture to it. Bake for 40 to 45 minutes, or until no longer runny, and serve.

VARIATION 1 **CRUSTLESS BROCCOLI-SAUSAGE TORTE:** Add ½ pound cooked Italian sausage to the broccoli mix.

VARIATION 2 **CRUSTLESS BROCCOLI TORTE WITH SUN-DRIED TOMATOES:** Add ½ cup chopped sun-dried tomatoes to the mix for a punch of concentrated flavor.

PREP TIP: If you're having trouble finding almond flour, you can make your own: Simply pulse 1 cup slivered almonds in a food processor until they reach a fine, flour-like consistency. Don't overprocess, or you'll end up with almond butter!

BROCCOLI WRAPS

This is a more involved recipe that gives you a great lunch option. Broccoli gets blended in the food processor and combined with eggs to make veggie-loaded lunch wraps with which you can wrap up sliced meat (or any filling, really) for a deliciously satisfying Paleo lunch. Wrap turkey and mayo, or even eggs and bacon, for an easy on-the-go breakfast. **SERVES 4**

PREP TIME: 15 minutes
COOK TIME: 20 minutes

1 head broccoli, cut into florets

3 eggs

3 garlic cloves, finely minced

1 shallot, minced

1 teaspoon chopped fresh chives

1 teaspoon dried oregano

1 teaspoon chopped
fresh parsley

1 teaspoon salt

Freshly ground black pepper

1. Preheat the oven to 350°F.

2. In a food processor or blender, pulse the broccoli until roughly chopped (don't overprocess—you want it to still be rough). Transfer to a microwave-safe bowl, and microwave on high for 2 minutes. Allow to cool for a few minutes, and then twist in a thin cloth or cheesecloth to remove any water (not a lot will come out, but the little that's there needs to be removed). Transfer the broccoli to a medium bowl.

3. In a small bowl, whisk together the eggs, garlic, shallot, chives, oregano, and parsley, and season with salt and pepper; pour over the broccoli, and mix until well incorporated.

4. Line a large baking sheet with parchment paper, and scoop the broccoli mixture into four equal sections. Spread each section of broccoli out until it's about ¼ inch thick, leaving a little room in between each. Bake for 10 minutes, and then flip and bake for another 7 minutes.

5. Remove the baking sheet from the oven, and allow the broccoli wraps to cool. Store in the refrigerator. To reheat, broil them quickly in the oven or toaster oven.

VARIATION 1 **TURKEY-AVOCADO BROCCOLI WRAP:** Layer 2 or 3 slices of turkey, a spread of Homemade Mayo (page 47), and ¼ avocado, sliced. Fold the wrap in half.

VARIATION 2 **BROCCOLI-WRAP TACOS:** Use the wraps as taco shells, and fill with Pulled Pork BBQ (page 74) or Blackened Shrimp (page 93).

PREP TIP: Make a large batch and freeze with parchment paper in between each wrap.

STEAMED BROCCOLI WITH HOLLANDAISE

Hollandaise is one of my favorite sauces, and probably the reason I order eggs Benedict any time I'm out to brunch. Often, I don't think to serve it over anything other than a poached egg, but broccoli does a great job holding up to hollandaise's buttery richness. I like to simply steam the broccoli while I mix up the hollandaise and then dip the broccoli into the sauce. **SERVES 4**

PREP TIME: 5 minutes
COOK TIME: 15 minutes

1 large head broccoli

4 egg yolks

1 tablespoon freshly squeezed lemon juice

½ cup unsalted, grass-fed butter (1 full stick), melted

¼ teaspoon ground cayenne pepper

Salt

1. In a steamer over boiling water, steam the broccoli for 4 to 5 minutes. If you don't have a steamer addition for your saucepan, you can boil the broccoli for 1 to 1½ minutes.

2. Bring a saucepan of water to a simmer. To make the hollandaise sauce, in a heatproof bowl that will fit over the saucepan (without the bottom touching the water), quickly whisk the egg yolks and lemon juice together until the mixture becomes frothy and starts to expand, about 30 seconds. Place the bowl over the saucepan, and continue to whisk. Slowly drizzle the melted butter in while stirring and continuing to whisk until the sauce has doubled in size, 3 to 4 minutes.

3. Remove from the heat, stir in the cayenne and a pinch of salt, and serve immediately or keep warm over a pan of warm (not hot) water until ready to serve.

VARIATION 1 **STEAMED BROCCOLI WITH CHIPOTLE HOLLANDAISE:** 1 tablespoon of the sauce from a can of chipotles in adobo sauce added to the hollandaise will give it a lovely smoky flavor.

VARIATION 2 **STEAMED ASPARAGUS WITH HOLLANDAISE:** Swap the broccoli for steamed asparagus. Follow the original recipe as written, but steam the asparagus for 6 to 8 minutes.

PALEO PAIR: Serve with Baked Tilapia or Salmon (page 81).

BACON-BROCCOLI BITES

These Paleo broccoli "bites" remind me a little bit of tater tots, except that instead of molding them into a tot shape, you simply drop them by the spoonful into a mini-muffin tin. I like them on their own as a snack, but if you've made them ahead of time, they also make a great breakfast on a busy morning. It's such an easy way to get extra veggies into your diet. **SERVES 4**

PREP TIME: 15 minutes
COOK TIME: 30 minutes

1 large head broccoli, cut into florets

1 onion, diced

3 garlic cloves, minced

3 slices bacon, cooked and chopped

3 eggs, whisked

Salt

Freshly ground black pepper

Coconut oil, for greasing

1. Preheat the oven to 350°F.

2. Bring a large saucepan of salted water to a boil. Add the broccoli florets, and cook for 5 minutes. Drain really well, and allow them to cool slightly.

3. In a food processor or blender, pulse the broccoli, onion, and garlic until pretty finely chopped, but stop before it turns into a purée. Transfer the mixture to a medium bowl, and stir to combine with the bacon and eggs. Season with salt and pepper.

4. Grease a mini-muffin tin with a paper towel dipped in coconut oil. Spoon the broccoli mixture into each muffin cup. If there's any leftover egg at the bottom of your bowl, pour it over the broccoli bites. Bake for 20 to 25 minutes, until set, and serve.

VARIATION 1 **BACON-BROCCOLI DROPS WITH RANCH:** Serve with a side of Ranch Dressing (page 75) as an appetizer.

VARIATION 2 **OLIVE-BROCCOLI DROPS:** For a vegetarian version, swap the bacon for ½ cup chopped Kalamata olives.

PREP TIP: Make these ahead of time and freeze. Defrost a few for breakfast or as appetizers when you're planning to entertain.

BROCCOLI-SWEET POTATO HASH

This recipe makes a great breakfast, lunch, or dinner dish and is complemented wonderfully by the addition of eggs (as you can see in the variation below). There's something so enduringly satisfying about the combination of sweet potato, sweet broccoli, and spicy chorizo. **SERVES 4**

PREP TIME: 10 minutes
COOK TIME: 20 minutes

30 **NF**

2 tablespoons grass-fed butter or ghee

½ onion, diced

1 garlic clove, minced

2 small sweet potatoes, peeled and diced

½ pound chorizo or Italian sausage

1 small head broccoli, finely chopped

1. In a large saucepan over medium heat, melt the butter. Sauté the onion and garlic until the onion is slightly translucent, about 5 minutes. Add the sweet potatoes, and cook for another 5 minutes.

2. Add the chorizo, break it up with a wooden spoon, and increase the heat to medium-high. Cook until the meat is no longer pink and bits of it begin to get crunchy and browned, another 5 minutes.

3. Add the broccoli and stir. Cook for 5 more minutes, and serve hot.

VARIATION 1 **BREAKFAST BROCCOLI HASH:** Serve with fried eggs. Crack them right into the pan you used for the hash, and cook on one side until the white is no longer runny. Carefully flip and cook for a minute or two on the other side, depending on how done you want the yolk.

VARIATION 2 **GROUND BEEF-BROCCOLI HASH:** Swap the chorizo or sausage for ground beef (the cook time should be about the same). Chorizo and Italian sausage are both on the spicy side, so swapping them out for ground beef will make this dish a bit milder.

PREP TIP: Dice your sweet potatoes as soon as you bring them home from the store; cutting them is often the most time-consuming part of any recipe that calls for sweet potatoes.

PANTRY STAPLE: HOMEMADE NUT BUTTER

Almond butter (and other nut butters) are such a great staple to have in your fridge—and you can easily make your own to ensure that you aren't consuming any hidden sugars or oils. I actually will make peanut butter for my dog (not Paleo, but neither is he!) this way because I hate to buy a big jar full of preservatives. I feel like homemade nut butter is the spirit of Paleo in a nutshell (forgive me for the pun, I couldn't help it): not a ton of work, and a whole lot of benefits. **MAKES ABOUT 2 CUPS**

PREP TIME: 15 minutes
COOK TIME: none

`30` `V`

2 cups raw almonds (or the nut of your choice)

1 to 2 tablespoons coconut oil

Combine all the ingredients in a food processor until the butter reaches the consistency you like (I prefer mine creamy but you could easily blend for less time and have chunky almond butter). This can take up to 15 minutes. Store in a jar in the refrigerator for up to two weeks.

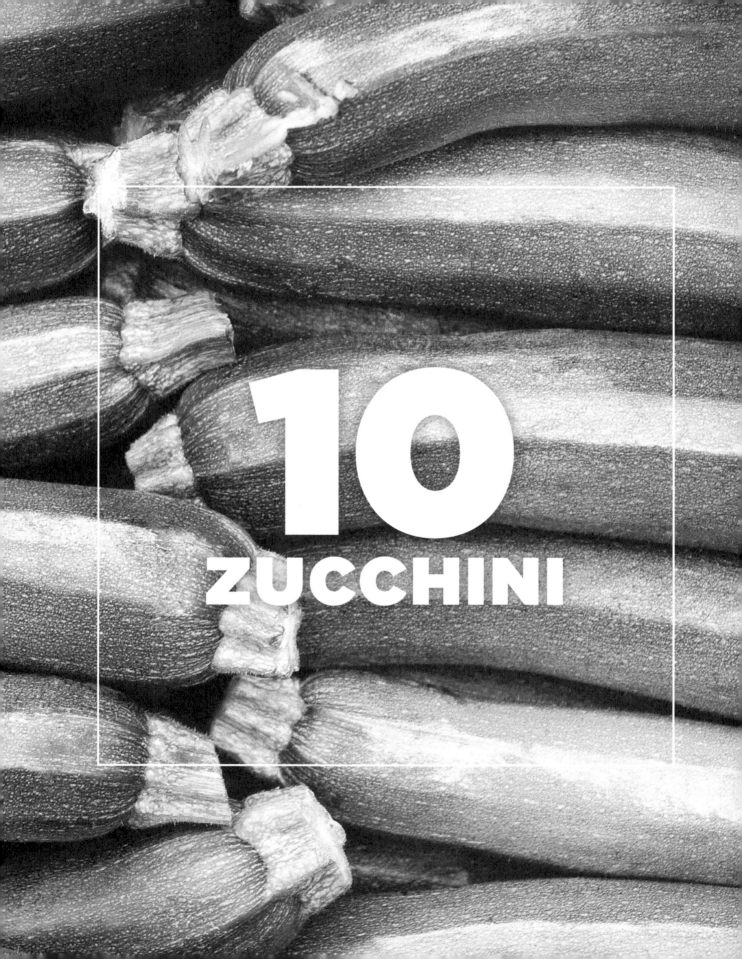

10
ZUCCHINI

I think Paleo eaters worldwide will agree that the discovery of zucchini noodles has absolutely changed their lives. When I first switched my diet, I didn't know how to give up pasta. I grew up in an Italian family, and we ate pasta with everything. For a long time I went without it, with the exception of some gluten-free pasta here and there when I felt like indulging without feeling too terrible later, but then I discovered the magic of zoodles, and how incredibly convincing spiralized zucchini can be at mimicking pasta!

Of course, there's more you can do with zucchini than turn it into a bowl of Paleo pasta—Baked Zucchini Fries (page 151), Zucchini Lasagna (page 155), and even one of the few things my grandma Angelica used to make for me as a child—Stuffed Zucchini Boats (page 157). I went back to my roots for this chapter, so I hope you love it.

ZUCCHINI-NOODLE SALAD WITH LEMON, PEAS, AND CASHEWS

This salad is incredibly light and refreshing—a perfect snack or light lunch for a warm afternoon. Zucchini noodles are perfect for salads; using the squash raw makes for a quick meal and a welcome variation from your usual leaf lettuce salads. This one is full of additional veggies like radishes and peas and seasoned with a splash of lemon and some homemade cashew cream. **SERVES 4**

PREP TIME: 10 minutes, plus 2 hours to soak
COOK TIME: None

V

½ cup raw cashews

½ cup water, plus more if necessary

Salt (optional)

Freshly ground black pepper (optional)

3 or 4 zucchini, spiralized or julienned into noodles

½ red bell pepper, diced

½ cup green peas (thawed if frozen)

2 or 3 radishes, sliced

¼ cup broccoli or broccolini florets

Juice of 1 lemon

½ lemon, sliced into wedges, for garnish

1. In a medium bowl, soak the cashews in the water for 2 hours, making sure there is enough water to cover them.

2. In a blender, blend the soaked cashews and soaking water to a creamy consistency. Season with salt and pepper (if using).

3. In a large bowl, stir well to combine the zucchini noodles, bell pepper, peas, radishes, broccoli, and lemon juice.

4. Plate the salad, drizzle with the cashew cream, garnish with lemon wedges, and serve.

VARIATION 1 **ZUCCHINI SALAD WITH LEMON, PEAS, AND SPICY CASHEW CREAM:** Spice up the cashew cream with ¼ teaspoon ground cayenne pepper. Taste and add more if you'd like it even hotter.

VARIATION 2 **SWEET POTATO NOODLES WITH LEMON, PEAS, AND CASHEW CREAM:** Spiralize 2 sweet potatoes, and sauté for 2 to 3 minutes over medium heat with 1 tablespoon olive oil. Remove from the heat, allow to cool slightly, and then assemble the rest of the salad according to the original recipe.

PREP TIP: Make the noodles the day before, and store in the refrigerator.

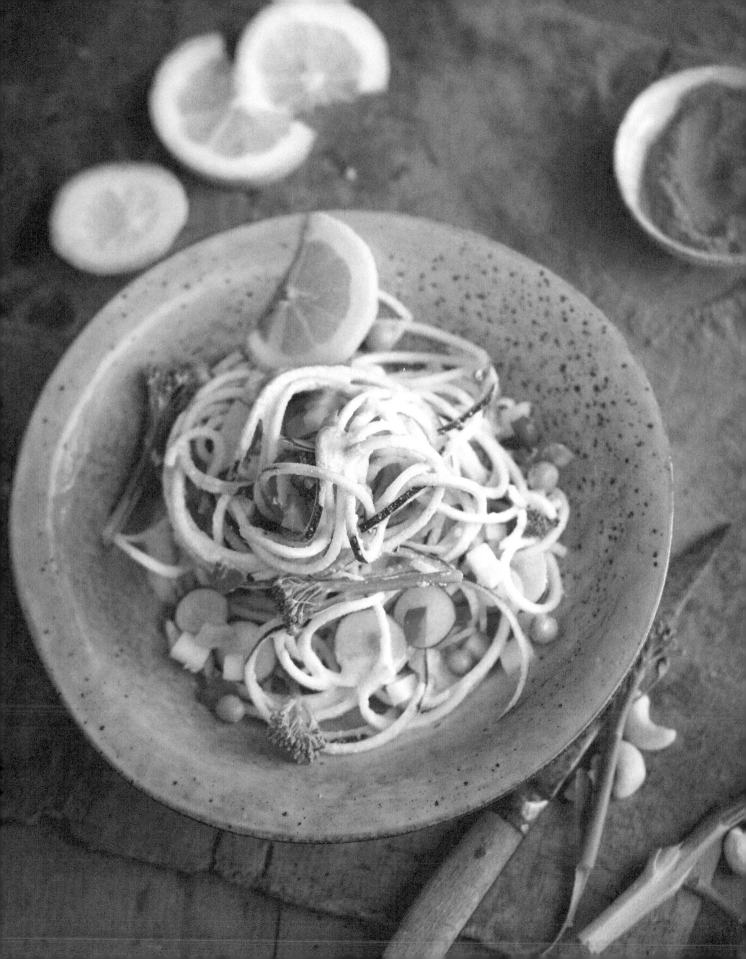

RATATOUILLE

Ratatouille is a classic vegetable dish that's pretty Paleo on its own—all I had to do to make it 100 percent was to skip the Parmesan cheese usually found sprinkled between the layers of vegetables. This dish can be as rustic or as fancy as you want; I've seen the layers tightly stacked in a circle around the baking dish so it looks almost like a kaleidoscope, and I've seen everything just thrown in and spooned out equally casually. Either way, the vegetables for this dish come together in a really delicious medley. **SERVES 4**

PREP TIME: 15 minutes
COOK TIME: 1 hour

`NF` `V`

2 tablespoons extra-virgin olive oil, divided

3 garlic cloves, minced

1 eggplant, diced

Salt

Freshly ground black pepper

2 teaspoons dried parsley

2 zucchini, cut into rounds

1 onion, cut into rings

1 green bell pepper, cut into strips

2 large tomatoes, chopped (or 10 ounces cherry tomatoes, sliced)

1 or 2 tablespoons chopped fresh parsley, for garnish

PREP TIP: Cut up all your veggies a day or two before. You can also assemble the dish ahead of time and then bake before serving (although you'll have to cook the eggplant the day of and put it on top instead of the bottom of the dish).

1. Preheat the oven to 350°F.

2. Grease a baking dish with 1 tablespoon of olive oil. In a large skillet over medium heat, heat the remaining 1 tablespoon of olive oil. Sauté the garlic until fragrant, about 2 minutes, and add the eggplant. Cook, stirring periodically, until the eggplant begins to soften, about 10 minutes. Season with salt, pepper, and the dried parsley.

3. Spread the eggplant across the bottom of a baking dish, and layer the zucchini rounds on top. Season with salt, and layer in the onion, bell pepper, and tomatoes, seasoning each layer with a pinch of salt and some pepper.

4. Bake for 45 minutes, until the vegetables are tender. Garnish with the fresh parsley and serve.

`VARIATION 1` **BREAKFAST RATATOUILLE:** Serve topped with one or two fried eggs for breakfast—just drizzle some olive oil into a hot skillet, and crack the egg gently over it. Cook on one side until the white is no longer runny. Carefully flip and cook for a minute or two on the other side, depending on how done you want the yolk.

`VARIATION 2` **RATATOUILLE WITH MUSHROOMS AND SAUSAGE:** Sauté 1 or 2 hot Italian sausages in a pan with 10 ounces mushrooms. Remove the sausage once it's cooked through, and slice. Add the mushroom-sausage mixture to the baking dish on top of the eggplant before layering on the remaining veggies and following the recipe as written.

BAKED ZUCCHINI FRIES

I grew up in Roanoke, Virginia, a little city; so if franchises like Starbucks came to town, it was always a Big Deal. When a Carrabba's Italian Grill opened in 2001, my high school girlfriends and I would go there for fun weekend lunches (it was next to the mall, after all). For some reason, it was only with my friend Emma that we'd order their fried zucchini appetizer—it was delicious and came with a tangy sauce I know now to be aioli. I wanted to make a Paleo version of zucchini fries that would capture both the delicious flavor and the sentimental memories I have of my best friends from high school. **SERVES 4 TO 6**

PREP TIME: 15 minutes
COOK TIME: 25 minutes

2 large zucchini

½ cup almond flour

1½ teaspoons garlic powder

1½ teaspoons onion powder

2 eggs, whisked

Salt

Freshly ground black pepper

1. Preheat the oven to 400°F.

2. Cut the ends off the zucchini, and cut them in half widthwise, then lengthwise. Cut into French fry-like strips, and pat dry with a paper towel.

3. In a small bowl, mix together the almond flour, garlic powder, and onion powder. Dip the zucchini fries in the egg, let any excess egg drip off, and toss them in the almond flour mixture. Season with salt and pepper.

4. Lay the fries out on a baking sheet, put them in the oven, and immediately lower the heat to 350°F. Cook for 20 to 25 minutes, or until the fries are crisp, checking on them halfway through the cooking time and lowering the heat if they're getting brown too quickly.

5. Serve immediately.

VARIATION 1 **CURLY ZUCCHINI FRIES:** Spiralize the zucchini and bake them the same way—but check on them after 7 minutes, since they'll be thinner.

VARIATION 2 **SPICY ZUCCHINI FRIES:** Add ¼ to ½ teaspoon red pepper flakes to the almond flour mixture.

PALEO PAIR: Serve these fries alongside Beef Tenderloin (page 56) for a Paleo take on steak frites, and mix Homemade Mayo (page 47) with ¼ teaspoon or so of garlic powder for a fantastic dipping sauce.

ZUCCHINI

PAD THAI

I can almost never say no to pad thai, but there's not very much that's Paleo about it. Sure, it's mostly gluten-free, but the peanut sauce and rice noodles don't make for a very primal-friendly meal. After a few too many orders of Thai takeout, I finally started experimenting at home and came up with this salad that's about as close to pad thai as I can imagine. **SERVES 4**

PREP TIME: 10 minutes
COOK TIME: 20 minutes

1 pound boneless skinless chicken breast

2 tablespoons coconut aminos

2 garlic cloves, minced

1 teaspoon grated fresh ginger

1 to 2 tablespoons almond butter

1 tablespoon freshly squeezed lime juice, plus 4 lime wedges for garnish

2 teaspoons fish sauce

¼ to ½ teaspoon red pepper flakes

2 large zucchini, spiralized or julienned into noodles

1 cup bean sprouts

⅓ cup slivered almonds

2 to 3 tablespoons chopped fresh cilantro, for garnish

1. In a large pot of water over high heat, boil or steam the chicken breasts for about 15 minutes, or until they're cooked through. Pat dry and slice into bite-size pieces.

2. In a large bowl, mix the coconut aminos, garlic, ginger, almond butter, lime juice, fish sauce, and red pepper flakes. Set aside.

3. In a large skillet over medium-low heat, gently sauté the zucchini noodles for 2 to 3 minutes, or until they just start to become tender. Remove from the heat, and mix in with the pad thai sauce. Stir in the chicken, and serve topped with bean sprouts, almonds, cilantro, and a wedge of lime.

VARIATION 1 **SHRIMP PAD THAI:** Swap the chicken breast for sautéed shrimp—about ½ to 1 pound.

VARIATION 2 **PAD THAI SALAD:** Serve this dish as more of a salad by leaving the zucchini raw and mixing it with ½ cup chopped romaine lettuce. Serve the sauce chilled as a salad dressing.

PREP TIP: Make the sauce ahead of time, and store in the refrigerator. Stir well before using.

ZUCCHINI-SPINACH FRITTERS

These spinach fritters are a specialty of my mom's, and I decided to make them with zucchini to add even more vegetables. They are super delicious as a snack, and they make a great breakfast with some eggs on the side. They're also really tasty with a dollop of Ranch Dressing (page 75), or you could make an aioli with Homemade Mayo (page 47) and a few cloves of roasted garlic (see page 101). **SERVES 4 TO 6**

PREP TIME: 5 minutes
COOK TIME: 10 to 15 minutes

1 (14-ounce) can artichoke hearts, drained and chopped

12 ounces fresh spinach, washed, cooked, and drained

1 large zucchini, shredded

6 scallions, chopped

2 or 3 garlic cloves, minced

2 eggs, lightly beaten

½ cup almond flour

1 teaspoon salt

1 tablespoon extra-virgin olive oil, plus more if needed

1. Using your hands, squeeze as much liquid out of the artichoke hearts, spinach, and zucchini as possible.

2. In a food processor or blender, pulse the artichoke hearts, spinach, zucchini, scallions, and garlic until roughly chopped. Transfer the mixture to a large bowl, add the eggs and almond flour, and season with salt. Mix well.

3. In a large nonstick sauté pan over medium-high heat, heat the olive oil. Drop heaping tablespoons of the mixture into the pan, and cook for 2 to 3 minutes on each side, flattening them a little with your spatula to make them into mini-pancake shapes.

4. Serve immediately.

VARIATION 1 **SPINACH-ARTICHOKE FRITTERS:** Skip the zucchini if you don't have any, and continue with the rest of the recipe as written.

VARIATION 2 **CARROT FRITTERS:** Swap the artichoke, spinach, and zucchini for 1 pound shredded carrots. These are just as fast to prepare but a bit sweeter.

PALEO PAIR: Serve these as an appetizer along with Dates Wrapped in Bacon (page 64) and Shrimp Kebabs (page 98).

EMERGENCY PASTA WITH ZOODLES

I grew up eating "Emergency Pasta," which is the nickname my grandpa Albino gave to the classic recipe more commonly known as *aglio, olio, e pepperoncini*, which most Italians have in their arsenal of quick recipes. My grandfather referred to it as Emergency Pasta because you always had the ingredients on hand; if someone came over unexpectedly, you could still make them a meal—because no one should ever leave your house hungry. **SERVES 4**

PREP TIME: 5 minutes
COOK TIME: 5 minutes

¼ cup extra-virgin olive oil

2 or 3 garlic cloves, thinly sliced

¼ hot red pepper, minced (or ¼ teaspoon red pepper flakes)

3 or 4 large zucchini, spiralized or julienned into noodles

Salt

Freshly ground black pepper

1. In a large sauté pan over medium-low heat, heat the olive oil. Add the garlic, and stir it around. Remove from the heat as soon as the garlic becomes fragrant—about 30 seconds—because you don't want to burn it at all. Add the hot red pepper, and pour the sauce into a serving dish.

2. In the same pan over medium heat, sauté the zucchini noodles for 3 to 4 minutes, just until slightly softened. Transfer the noodles to the serving dish, season with salt and pepper, and toss with the sauce.

3. Serve immediately.

VARIATION 1 **EMERGENCY PASTA WITH CHICKEN:** Make this dish a little heartier by adding diced chicken to the pan. Add an extra tablespoon of olive oil and a few more pinches of salt.

VARIATION 2 **PESTO ZOODLES:** Make the zucchini noodles according to the recipe above, and then dress them with Pesto (page 175) instead of *aglio, olio, e pepperoncini*.

PALEO PAIR: Serve as a side with Shrimp Kebabs (page 98).

ZUCCHINI LASAGNA

This uses lasagna zucchini instead of pasta. The beef, sausage, and thick tomato sauce are so satisfying in themselves that no one will be complaining.

SERVES 6 TO 8

PREP TIME: 15 minutes
COOK TIME: 1 hour, 30 minutes

DF **NF**

2 large zucchini

1 pound spicy Italian sausage

1 pound ground beef

1 onion, diced

1 small green bell pepper, diced

1 (16-ounce) can tomato sauce

1 cup tomato paste

¼ cup red wine (optional; omit if strict Paleo)

2 tablespoons chopped fresh basil

2 tablespoons chopped fresh parsley

1 tablespoon chopped fresh oregano

Salt

Freshly ground black pepper

1 pound fresh mushrooms, sliced

PREP TIP: Cook the meat and assemble the lasagna ahead of time. Store in the refrigerator and bake about 1½ hours before you're ready to serve it.

1. Preheat the oven to 325°F.

2. Use a vegetable peeler to cut the zucchini lengthwise into small, thin sheets that resemble lasagna.

3. In a large skillet over medium heat, cook the Italian sausage for 5 to 7 minutes per side, until browned. Remove from the skillet, and set aside. Add the ground beef to the skillet, and cook for 5 minutes, using a wooden spoon to break up the beef. Add the onion and bell pepper, and continue cooking until the beef is no longer pink, about another 5 minutes.

4. Stir in the tomato sauce, tomato paste, wine (if using), basil, parsley, and oregano, and season with salt and pepper. Once the sauce begins to boil, reduce the heat and simmer for 20 minutes, stirring frequently. Remove from the heat.

5. To assemble the lasagna, start by spreading half the meat sauce into the bottom of an 8-by-12-inch baking dish. Layer half the zucchini slices over the meat sauce. Add the Italian sausage and all the mushrooms. Continue layering the lasagna by adding the remaining meat sauce and zucchini sheets.

6. Cover with foil, and bake the lasagna for 45 minutes. Carefully remove the foil, raise the oven temperature to 375°F, and bake for an additional 10 to 15 minutes.

7. Remove from the oven and allow to rest for 5 minutes before slicing. Serve warm.

VARIATION 1 **ZUCCHINI-SPINACH LASAGNA:** Add a layer of cooked spinach to the lasagna—wash 12 ounces spinach well, quickly boil and drain it (or use precooked frozen spinach, thawed), and layer it over the Italian sausage.

VARIATION 2 **PIZZA LASAGNA:** Add a layer of pepperoni to the zucchini and serve with a side of sugar-free marinara sauce (Traders Joe's marina sauce in the big green can is my favorite Paleo-friendly brand).

ZUCCHINI-NOODLE RAMEN

I grew up eating the instant kind of ramen in the orange package. I loved it plain, but my dad and brother would always add stuff to it, which I eventually grew to appreciate as I discovered all the awesome things you can put in it. I've definitely missed ramen as I've experimented with my gluten sensitivity over the years, so sometimes I'll make it with gluten-free noodles, but this recipe is Paleo-friendly and, with the substitution of zucchini noodles, completely grain free. **SERVES 4 TO 6**

PREP TIME: 20 minutes, plus overnight to chill
COOK TIME: 2 hours, 30 minutes

DF **NF**

1 pound pork tenderloin

1 tablespoon salt

2 bunches scallions, divided

1 (1-inch) piece fresh ginger root, sliced

4 garlic cloves, crushed

Toppings (optional): hardboiled eggs, kimchi, jalapeño peppers, fresh cilantro

5 tablespoons coconut aminos

2 tablespoons sake (optional; omit if strict Paleo)

1½ tablespoons sesame oil

4 large zucchini, spiralized or julienned

1. Season the pork with the salt, and refrigerate overnight.

2. Remove the pork from the refrigerator, and place in a large saucepan over medium-high heat. Add 1½ bunches of scallions and the ginger and garlic to the pan with enough water to just cover the pork. Bring to a boil, lower the heat, and simmer for at least 2 hours (although longer is better, if possible).

3. While the broth is cooking, prepare all your toppings (if using): Soft-boil the eggs (see page 31), slice the jalapeños and the remaining ½ bunch of scallions, and chop the cilantro.

4. Add the coconut aminos, sake (if using), and sesame oil to the broth. Continue to simmer, and add the zucchini noodles about 5 minutes before you're ready to serve.

5. Transfer the pork to a platter, slice it, and transfer it back to the saucepan. Serve the ramen with whichever toppings sound good to you.

VARIATION 1 **ZUCCHINI-NOODLE CHICKEN RAMEN:** Make this recipe with 1 pound chicken thighs or breasts instead of the pork. Continue with the recipe as written.

VARIATION 2 **SQUASH-NOODLE RAMEN:** Instead of spiralized zucchini, use a vegetable peeler to create thin, wide squash noodles. Continue with the recipe as written.

PREP TIP: Season the pork and make the broth in advance so all you'll have to do is heat everything together. This will save you one night of prep as well as a couple of hours of simmering.

STUFFED ZUCCHINI BOATS

My grandma Angelica was not much of a cook, but she made a few things that were awesome: *arroz con leche*, crepes (still referred to as "grandma pancakes" in our family), saltine crackers with butter and sugar (as complicated as it sounds, but truly delicious and an afternoon snack that became a tradition with my college roommate), and these stuffed zucchini boats. **SERVES 4**

PREP TIME: 10 minutes
COOK TIME: 1 hour

4 large zucchini

1 pound ground beef

2 tablespoons extra-virgin olive oil

1 onion, diced

2 garlic cloves, chopped

Salt

Freshly ground black pepper

¾ cup green olives, roughly chopped

2 hardboiled eggs, chopped

1. Preheat the oven to 350°F.

2. Cut the zucchini lengthwise, and scoop the insides out with a spoon. Chop the inside parts, and add them to a medium bowl with the ground beef.

3. In a large skillet over medium-high heat, heat the olive oil. Sauté the onion and garlic until the onion is slightly translucent, about 5 minutes. Add the ground beef-zucchini mixture, and cook for about 5 minutes more, until completely browned, breaking the meat up as you cook it. Season with salt and pepper.

4. Remove the skillet from the heat, and add the olives and hard-boiled eggs. Stir well.

5. Stuff the zucchini boats with the meat mixture, and place them on a baking sheet. Bake for 45 minutes, until tender, and serve.

VARIATION 1 **STUFFED BELL PEPPERS:** Cut the tops off 4 green or red bell peppers, and remove and discard the seeds and membranes. Stuff with the meat mixture, and bake at 350°F for 45 minutes.

VARIATION 2 **TURKEY-STUFFED ZUCCHINI BOATS:** Swap ground beef for ground turkey for a lighter version, and follow the recipe as written.

PREP TIP: Assemble the zucchini boats the day before and bake before serving.

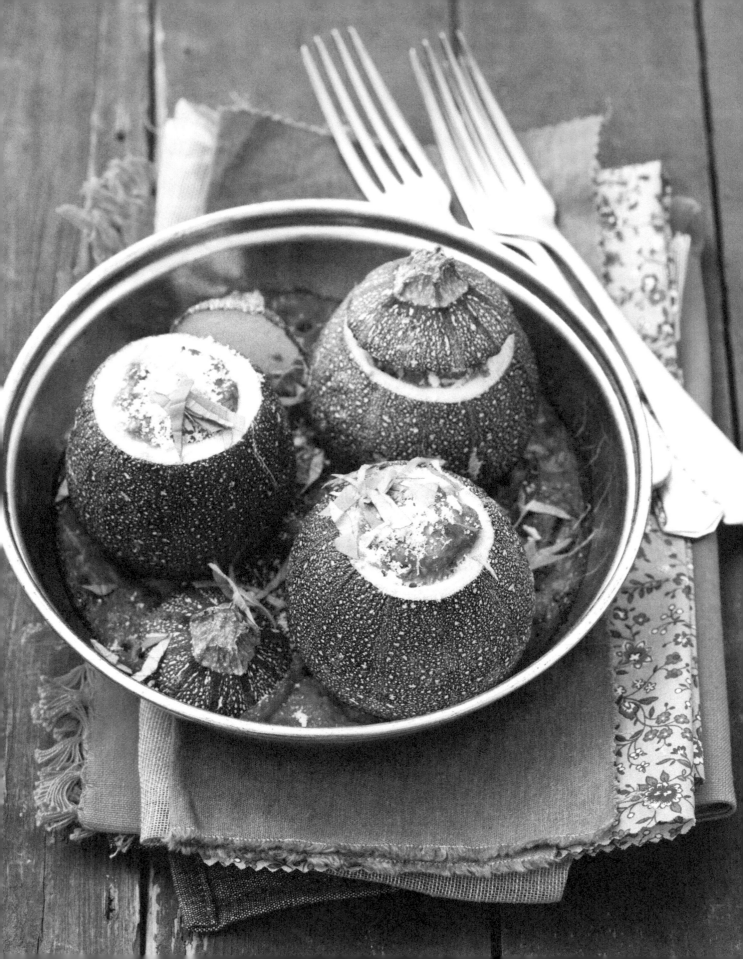

STUFFED SQUASH

I make this stuffed squash all the time in the fall and winter—it tastes great and seems pretty fancy even though it doesn't take much time or effort to pull off. You can make these with any round squash you like; so far, my favorite is acorn. The first time I made this, my husband and I were living in Minnesota; it was our first winter there together, and roasted squash stuffed with savory meat in tomato sauce just felt right. **SERVES 2**

PREP TIME: 10 minutes
COOK TIME: 1 hour

2 round squash, such as acorn or 8-ball zucchini

2 tablespoons extra-virgin olive oil

Salt

Freshly ground black pepper

½ teaspoon onion powder

½ onion, diced

1 pound ground beef

1½ teaspoons garlic powder

1½ teaspoons dried oregano

⅛ teaspoon red pepper flakes

1 (14.5-ounce) can diced tomatoes, drained

1 or 2 tablespoons chopped fresh basil or oregano

1. Preheat the oven to 350°F.

2. Carefully cut the tops off the squash, scoop out the seeds, trim the bottoms if necessary so they will stand up straight, and season the insides with the olive oil, salt, pepper, and onion powder. Roast for 45 minutes.

3. While the squash are in the oven, in a large sauté pan over medium heat, sauté the onion until slightly translucent, about 5 minutes. Add the beef, and break it up with a wooden spoon. Season with the garlic powder, oregano, red pepper flakes, and some more salt and pepper.

4. Once the beef is no longer pink, 7 to 8 minutes, reduce the heat to low and add the tomatoes. Continue to simmer until the squash have finished cooking.

5. To serve, place each squash in a bowl or on a plate and spoon the beef mixture into the centers. Garnish with the basil.

VARIATION 1 **STUFFED ONION:** Cut an onion in half, and remove most of the inside. Stuff each half with the ground beef mixture, and bake at 350°F for 20 minutes.

VARIATION 2 **SPICY STUFFED SQUASH:** To kick up the heat a notch, use 1 pound hot Italian sausage instead of beef (the cook time may be a few minutes longer).

PREP TIP: Assemble the stuffed squash up to 1 day ahead of time, and reheat when ready to serve.

ZUCCHINI-NOODLE LO MEIN

When my family moved from the San Francisco Bay Area to Roanoke, Virginia, we were surprised to find that what we had always referred to as "chow mein" was actually called "lo mein." Maybe it's a regional difference, but whatever you call it, this is a Paleo version made with zucchini, and it satisfies my very regular cravings for a big bowl of sweet and salty crunchy Asian noodles, without having to succumb to expensive and not-so-healthy takeout. **SERVES 4**

PREP TIME: 10 minutes
COOK TIME: 20 minutes

30 **NF** **V**

2 tablespoons sesame oil

½ onion, diced

2 garlic cloves, minced

¼ teaspoon grated fresh ginger

1 red bell pepper, finely diced

2 large carrots, finely chopped

¼ teaspoon chili oil or chili paste

2 tablespoons coconut aminos

4 large zucchini, spiralized or julienned into noodles

½ cup green peas (thawed if frozen)

2 tablespoons sesame seeds, for garnish

1 or 2 tablespoons sliced scallions, for garnish

1. In a large skillet over medium heat, heat the sesame oil. Sauté the onion, garlic, and ginger until the onion is slightly translucent, about 5 minutes. Add the bell pepper and carrots, and sauté for another 5 minutes.

2. Add the chili oil and coconut aminos. Stir everything well, and add the zucchini noodles. Sauté for another 2 to 3 minutes, and add the green peas. Cook for a final 3 to 4 minutes, and then remove from the heat.

3. Garnish with the sesame seeds and scallions, and serve.

VARIATION 1 **PALEO CHICKEN LO MEIN:** Sauté 2 diced chicken breasts with the onion, garlic, and ginger (the cook time should be about the same if diced small enough). Continue with the rest of the recipe as written.

VARIATION 2 **SHRIMP LO MEIN:** Add 1 pound peeled, deveined shrimp to the pan with the onion, garlic, and ginger, and cook until the shrimp turn pink (the cook time should be about the same). Continue with the rest of the recipe as written.

PREP TIP: Chop all your veggies and spiralize the zucchini ahead of time so all you'll have to do is sauté.

PANTRY BASIC: BLACKENING SPICE MIX

This blackening spice mix is especially good on shrimp and other seafood—when you use it, make sure the protein of choice is patted dry, and then toss it thoroughly in a bowl with the spice mix. You want to make sure it's well covered, like you were breading something before you fry it. Then cook in a dry, hot pan. **MAKES ¼ CUP**

PREP TIME: 5 minutes
COOK TIME: None

30 **NF** **V**

2 teaspoons chili powder

2 teaspoons garlic powder

2 teaspoons ground paprika

1 teaspoon ground allspice

1 teaspoon onion powder

1 teaspoon dried oregano

1 teaspoon red pepper flakes

1 teaspoon salt

1 teaspoon dried thyme

½ teaspoon dried basil

½ teaspoon ground cayenne pepper

½ teaspoon freshly ground black pepper

½ teaspoon white pepper

In a mason jar or other container with a tightly fitting lid, mix or shake to combine the chili powder, garlic powder, paprika, allspice, onion powder, oregano, red pepper flakes, salt, thyme, basil, cayenne pepper, and black and white pepper.

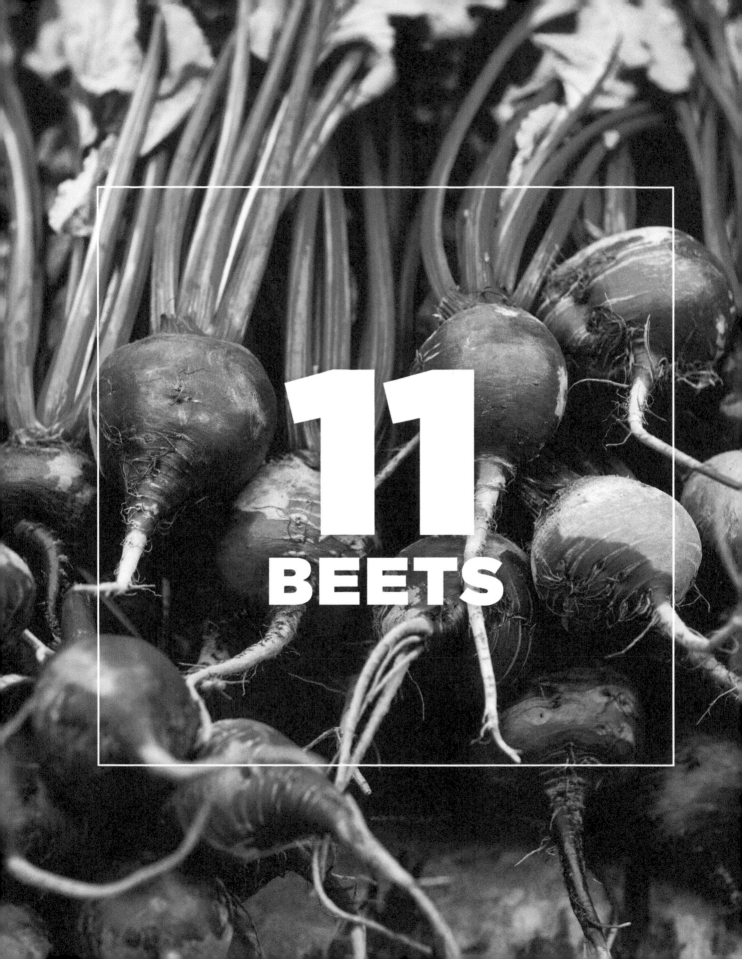

11
BEETS

Beets can make a mess—my tips for handling that are to peel them in the sink and make sure you cut them on a surface that's easy to wipe, not at all porous, and won't stain (think plastic cutting board, not wooden). I like using beets with orange or lemon because they have a really nice naturally sweet quality that is enhanced by the citrus, but they're also delicious roasted with some salt and pepper, and they're a great variation from sweet potatoes or other root vegetables.

Some of these recipes feel kind of like treats—the Ginger-Beet Sorbet (page 172) is delicious, and the bright pink Beet Lemonade (page 171) is perfect for a hot afternoon. This chapter is definitely the most unusual, because beets themselves are a little unusual, so have fun branching out and experimenting!

ROASTED BEETS

Roasting beets seems to be the most common way of preparing the little red root veggies, and for good reason—it's a tasty, easy way of cooking them. A few of the recipes in this chapter begin with roasted beets, so it only makes sense to start with a basic recipe for roasting. You can season them any way you want, but a great neutral start is with olive oil, salt, and pepper.

SERVES 4 TO 6

PREP TIME: 10 minutes
COOK TIME: 40 minutes

8 beets, peeled and cut into chunks

2 tablespoons extra-virgin olive oil

Salt

Freshly ground black pepper

1. Preheat the oven to 400°F.

2. On a baking sheet, spread out the chunks of beet and drizzle with the olive oil. Season with salt and pepper, and use your hands to mix it all together.

3. Bake for 35 to 40 minutes, checking on them halfway through the cooking time and mixing with a spatula.

4. Serve warm.

VARIATION 1 **ORANGE-GINGER ROASTED BEETS:** Season the beets with ½ teaspoon dried ginger. When you remove the beets from the oven, squeeze the juice of ½ orange over them.

VARIATION 2 **BALSAMIC-ROASTED BEETS:** Add 1 or 2 tablespoons balsamic vinegar to the beets before roasting. Adding balsamic vinegar creates a wonderfully sweet balance of tanginess.

PALEO PAIR: Serve these roasted beets with Prosciutto-Wrapped Chicken Thighs (page 45).

BEET AND CITRUS SALAD

The flavor combination of beets and citrus is fabulous, so this salad of roasted beets loaded with oranges and grapefruit dressed with a simple lemon vinaigrette is a winner. You could serve it over greens or just scoop it into bowls on its own. **SERVES 4**

PREP TIME: 15 minutes
COOK TIME: 40 minutes

6 beets, peeled and cut into chunks

3 tablespoons extra-virgin olive oil, divided

Salt

Freshly ground black pepper

1 orange, peeled and cut into segments

1 grapefruit, peeled and cut into segments

Juice of 1 lemon

Several fresh mint leaves, for garnish

1. Preheat the oven to 400°F.

2. On a baking sheet, spread out the chunks of beet and drizzle with 1½ tablespoons of olive oil. Season with salt and pepper, and use your hands to mix it all together.

3. Bake for 35 to 40 minutes, checking on them halfway through the cooking time and mixing with a spatula. Remove and cool completely.

4. In a large bowl, mix the beets with the orange and grapefruit sections. Dress with the remaining 1½ tablespoons of olive oil and the lemon juice, and give it a good stir. Garnish with the fresh mint leaves and serve.

VARIATION 1 **BEET AND CITRUS SALAD WITH PISTACHIOS:** Top the salad with ¼ cup crushed pistachios for a pop of green, a nice crunch, and a dose of healthy fats.

VARIATION 2 **BEET AND CITRUS SALAD WITH TURMERIC (OR CUMIN):** Add ¼ teaspoon turmeric (or cumin, if preferred) to the salad. Turmeric has a slight gingery taste that goes really well with beets.

PREP TIP: Roast your beets and section the citrus (store in the refrigerator) ahead of time so when it's time to serve the salad, you'll just need a few minutes to assemble.

BEET-NOODLE SALAD

This salad is all about the beets—while the recipe calls for a few greens, they're mostly for garnish. These raw beet-and-radish noodles are tender and sweet and so delicious tossed in your favorite dressing. Serve them on their own or with the protein of your choice to take it from snack or side dish to complete meal. **SERVES 2**

PREP TIME: 15 minutes
COOK TIME: None

1 red beet, spiralized

1 golden beet, spiralized

1 or 2 watermelon radishes, spiralized

¼ cup microgreens (or your favorite salad green)

2 tablespoons Balsamic Vinaigrette (page 89) or cashew cream (see page 148)

Salt

Freshly ground black pepper

1. In a serving bowl, toss to combine the red beet, golden beet, and radish noodles with the greens.

2. Add the Balsamic Vinaigrette or cashew cream (or 2 tablespoons of your favorite Paleo salad dressing), and toss again. Season with salt and pepper and serve.

VARIATION 1 **BEET-NOODLE SALAD WITH SHRIMP:** Top the salad with 5 to 6 ounces Blackened Shrimp (page 93).

VARIATION 2 **BEET-NOODLE SALAD WITH AVOCADO:** Top the salad with ½ diced avocado and a squeeze of lime juice.

PREP TIP: If you don't have a spiralizer, you can use a vegetable peeler to get long, thin ribbons, and then slice them thinly. (Some vegetable peelers have a julienne side; if that's the case, use that and skip the slicing.)

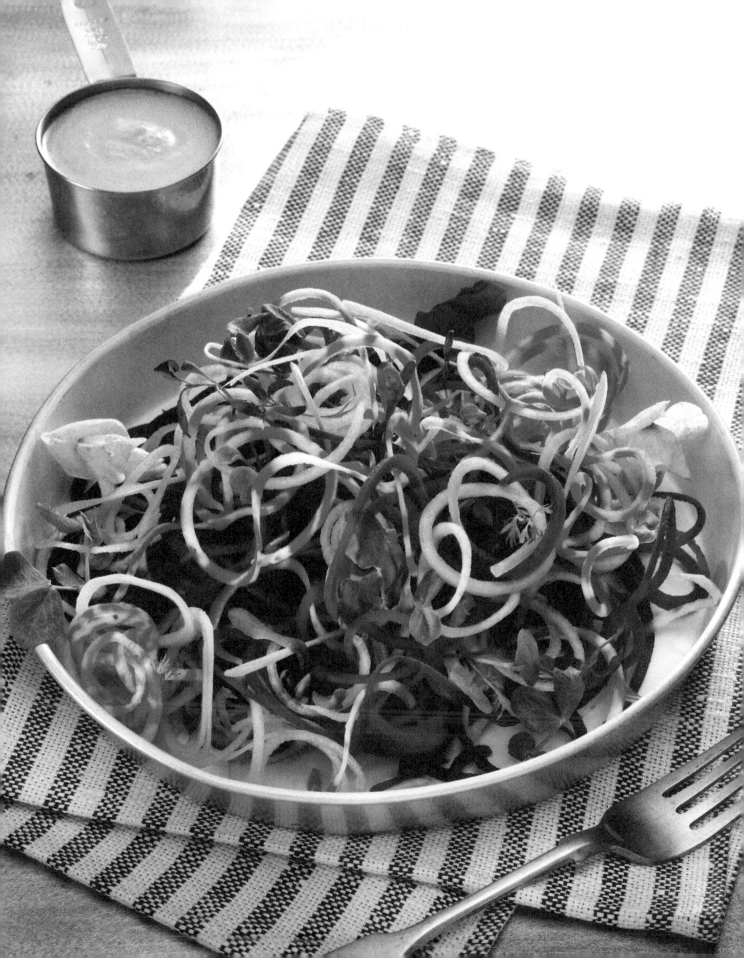

BORSCHT

Borscht is such a wonderfully tasty way to use up any veggies you might have in your refrigerator. The combination of beets and fresh dill is great, and the beef broth gives the soup a lovely richness. You can make your own beef broth (see the Chicken Soup recipe, page 36), but if you're in a hurry or don't have any, some store-bought broth will do the trick. **SERVES 4**

PREP TIME: 15 minutes
COOK TIME: 40 minutes

8 cups beef broth

2 tablespoons extra-virgin olive oil

1 onion, diced

2 garlic cloves, minced

2 carrots, chopped

2 celery stalks, chopped

1 teaspoon dried oregano

Salt

Freshly ground black pepper

2 dried bay leaves

3 beets, peeled

¼ cup minced fresh dill

2 tablespoons red wine vinegar

1. In a medium saucepan over medium-high heat, bring the broth to a boil. Reduce the heat to low, and simmer.

2. In a large saucepan over medium heat, heat the olive oil. Sauté the onion and garlic until the onion becomes slightly translucent, about 5 minutes.

3. Add the carrots, celery, and oregano to the onions and garlic, season with salt and pepper, and stir. Reduce the heat to low, and cook for 7 to 8 minutes, or until the vegetables become fork-tender.

4. Carefully transfer the simmering broth to the pot with the vegetables. Add the bay leaves, and continue to simmer for about 10 minutes.

5. Grate the beets right into the soup, and simmer for an additional 15 minutes.

6. Add the dill, and remove the borscht from the heat. Stir in the red wine vinegar and serve.

VARIATION 1 **VEGETARIAN BORSCHT:** Use vegetable broth instead of beef broth if you'd like to make a vegetarian-friendly soup.

VARIATION 2 **BORSCHT WITH COCONUT CREAM:** Traditionally, borscht is served garnished with sour cream, but since dairy isn't Paleo, you can top it with whipped coconut cream—refrigerate a can of coconut cream overnight and then scoop the solid part out from the top. Whip it quickly in a mixer to make it extra fluffy, and season with salt, pepper, and garlic powder to bring out a more savory flavor. Spoon a dollop onto the soup.

PREP TIP: Make this soup ahead of time, and reheat on the stove before serving.

PICKLED BEETS

I absolutely love all pickles—cucumbers, okra, carrots, cauliflower—so if you can pickle it, I will probably eat it. It was only a matter of time before I started making my own. These pickled beets are delicious and make a great snack, and you can use the brine on any vegetable you want. My husband isn't a pickle fan like I am, but when they're homemade (and especially quick-pickled like these), he actually quite enjoys them. So make a batch for the pickle-cautious people in your life, and see how it goes—or you can just eat them all yourself. **SERVES 4 TO 6**

PREP TIME: 10 minutes
COOK TIME: 5 minutes
TOTAL TIME: 24 hours, 15 minutes

DF NF

½ cup red wine vinegar (or plain white vinegar)

½ cup water

5 whole peppercorns

2 or 3 whole cloves

2 dried bay leaves

2 tablespoons honey

2 or 3 beets, thinly sliced

1. In a medium saucepan over medium-high heat, bring the vinegar, water, peppercorns, cloves, bay leaves, and honey to a boil. Reduce the heat to low, and simmer for about 5 minutes. Remove from the heat.

2. Place the sliced beets in a wide-mouthed jar or other container, and carefully pour the liquid over them until they're covered by about an inch. Let them come to room temperature, and then refrigerate for at least 24 hours before serving.

VARIATION 1 **PICKLED BEET SALAD:** Add ½ cup pickled beets to a bowl with 1½ cups of your favorite salad greens. Top with crushed walnuts or almonds.

VARIATION 2 **BURGER BOWLS WITH PICKLED BEETS:** Use these pickles as a topping on your next Burger Bowls (page 51), or make Marinated Portobello Mushrooms (page 210) and top them with the pickled beets.

PREP TIP: These will last in the refrigerator for 7 to 10 days, so make them ahead of time if you're planning to serve them later.

BEET HUMMUS

I was never a big fan of hummus, so I didn't feel like I was missing out when I found out that regular hummus isn't Paleo (chickpeas are a legume, like peanuts, so they aren't included in the diet). This Paleo hummus is made out of beets, which I love, and the color is just gorgeous. Beet and lemon is a fantastic flavor combination, as you'll see not only for this recipe but also the fun Beet Lemonade recipe (page 171). **SERVES 4 TO 6**

PREP TIME: 15 minutes
COOK TIME: None

3 or 4 Roasted Beets (page 164)

1 small garlic clove

½ cup freshly squeezed lemon juice

Generous drizzle extra-virgin olive oil

Salt

Freshly ground black pepper

Raw vegetables of your choice, for serving

1. In a food processor or blender, pulse the Roasted Beets, garlic, lemon juice, and olive oil until smooth. Season with salt and pepper.

2. Serve with raw vegetables like carrots, celery, and sliced cucumber.

VARIATION 1 **SESAME-BEET HUMMUS:** Add 1 to 2 tablespoons tahini paste to the mix, and garnish with a sprinkle of sesame seeds.

VARIATION 2 **BEET HUMMUS WRAP:** Spread 2 or 3 tablespoons beet hummus on a romaine leaf or butter lettuce cup. Add a shredded carrot and a few cucumber slices. Wrap it up and enjoy as a light lunch or snack.

PALEO PAIR: Serve with Sweet Potato Fries (page 218).

BEET LEMONADE

This beet lemonade sounds a little unusual but is super delicious and refreshing—I love the bright pink color, and the sweetness of the beets lends itself to the lemonade so you don't have to use a ton of sweetener. I like it with just a little honey, garnished with a sprig of fresh mint. **SERVES 4 TO 6**

PREP TIME: 10 minutes
COOK TIME: 10 minutes
TOTAL TIME: 1 hour, 20 minutes

1 medium beet, peeled and grated

1 cup freshly squeezed lemon juice (about 4 or 5 large lemons)

3½ cups water

½ cup honey (or more, depending on how sweet you want it)

1. In a blender, blend the beet, lemon juice, water, and honey. Pour through a fine strainer into a pitcher. Use a spoon to press down on the beet pulp to strain out as much liquid as possible, and discard the pulp.

2. Chill for about an hour, and serve over lots of ice.

VARIATION 1 **STRAWBERRY-BEET LEMONADE:** Add 1 cup strawberries to the blender with the rest of the ingredients.

VARIATION 2 **LIME-BEET LEMONADE:** Follow the recipe as written, and then add 1 or 2 sliced limes to the pitcher in the refrigerator.

PREP TIP: Make a double batch of this lemonade and store in the refrigerator, or freeze in ice cube trays for later.

GINGER-BEET SORBET

Sometimes I really need a treat in the middle of the afternoon or after dinner, but finding Paleo-friendly desserts can be tricky. Every now and again, I'll buy a pint of almond or coconut milk ice cream, but those are still full of sugar and preservatives; This ginger-beet sorbet, however, is perfect, and it only takes a few ingredients. **SERVES 4**

PREP TIME: 10 minutes
COOK TIME: 30 minutes
TOTAL TIME: 1 hour, 40 minutes

2 or 3 beets, peeled and chopped into small chunks

1 cup water

Zest of 1 orange

¼ cup honey

½ teaspoon minced fresh ginger (or ¼ teaspoon dried)

Juice of 4 oranges

1. In a medium saucepan over medium-high heat, bring the beets, water, orange zest, honey, and ginger to a boil. Reduce the heat to low, and simmer for 20 to 30 minutes, until the beets are tender.

2. Pour the mixture into a blender, and blend until puréed. Allow to cool slightly (you can refrigerate for an hour), and then stir in the orange juice.

3. Use an ice cream maker if you have one; otherwise, just pour the liquid into a container with a lid, freeze until it reaches your desired consistency (I like mine just a little slushy), and serve.

VARIATION 1 **STRAWBERRY-RHUBARB SORBET:** Swap the beets for rhubarb and cook the same way, following the recipe as written, but leave out the orange juice, blend 6 ounces strawberries, and add them when you would add the orange juice. The minced ginger is optional for this version.

VARIATION 2 **LIME-BEET SORBET:** Swap the orange zest and juice for lime. Add an additional 2 to 3 tablespoons honey to balance out the tangy lime.

PREP TIP: Make a double batch of this and keep it in your freezer—you can let it defrost to the right consistency whenever you're in the mood for a cold treat.

BEET CHIPS

Root vegetable chips are really popular among the Paleo community, but they are very expensive to buy in a grocery store. Making them yourself is not only easy but also a lot more Paleo-friendly, because you can control exactly what goes into them—in this case, just beets, olive oil, and salt. **SERVES 2 TO 4**

PREP TIME: 10 minutes
COOK TIME: 20 minutes

3 beets

1 tablespoon extra-virgin olive oil

Salt

1. Preheat the oven to 350°F.

2. Scrub the beets, and cut the ends off. Use a mandolin (if you have one) to slice them into thin coins. Transfer the beet chips to a medium bowl, and season with the olive oil and salt. Spread them out into an even layer on a baking sheet, and bake for 20 minutes.

3. Remove from the oven and allow to cool right on the baking sheet—they'll crisp up a bit as they do—and serve.

VARIATION 1 **PARSNIP CHIPS:** Slice 1 parsnip in the mandolin, and follow the rest of the recipe as written. Parsnip chips will have a flavor and texture similar to a carrot, and perhaps even a bit sweeter.

VARIATION 2 **TARO ROOT CHIPS:** If you can find them, follow this recipe with taro root. Taro root is on the nuttier side, and it's one of my favorite vegetables to make chips with (I'm a big fan of those Terra brand taro root chips you can find at the store).

PALEO PAIR: Serve for lunch as a side with Broccoli Wraps (page 141) filled with turkey.

GOLDEN BEETS WITH BLUEBERRY VINAIGRETTE

Believe it or not, this dish originated when my brother created it for a Valentine's Day tasting menu for his sweet girlfriend, Jane. Beets with blueberries is definitely an unusual combination, especially when the berries are incorporated into a vinaigrette, but I'm pretty sure you'll enjoy it. Make it for someone special soon—they'll love it too. **SERVES 4**

PREP TIME: 10 minutes
COOK TIME: 45 minutes

30 NF V

2 or 3 golden beets

¼ onion, sliced

2 garlic cloves, minced

2 dried bay leaves

¼ teaspoon whole allspice

¼ teaspoon whole cloves

¼ teaspoon cumin seeds

¼ teaspoon mustard seeds

2 tablespoons fresh blueberries, plus more for garnish

¼ cup Balsamic Vinaigrette (page 89)

Salt

Freshly ground black pepper

3 or 4 fresh basil leaves, chopped

1. In a medium saucepan over medium-high heat, bring the beets, onion, garlic, bay leaves, allspice, cloves, cumin seeds, mustard seeds, and enough water to cover the beets to a boil. Cook until fork-tender, about 45 minutes. Drain and allow to cool.

2. In a small bowl, muddle the blueberries, mashing them with a spoon, and mix well with the Balsamic Vinaigrette.

3. Dice the beets, and toss with the blueberry-balsamic vinaigrette. Season with salt and pepper, garnish with more blueberries and the fresh basil, and serve.

VARIATION 1 **GOLDEN BEET SALAD WITH BLUEBERRY VINAIGRETTE:** Serve the beets on top of 1 cup field greens, arugula, or chopped romaine lettuce.

VARIATION 2 **RED BEETS WITH BLUEBERRY VINAIGRETTE:** Make this recipe with red beets if you can't find golden beets or prefer the red ones.

PREP TIP: Cook the beets ahead of time and refrigerate until ready to serve.

PANTRY BASIC: PESTO

My mom is known for her awesome pesto. We used to have pasta with pesto all the time when I was younger, but now that we're Paleo we like to serve it on chicken, shrimp, and even salads. The original recipe had Parmesan cheese in it, but we simply skip it and you can barely tell the difference. It freezes really well (I used to bring pounds of it to college with me), so make a double batch and save some for later. **MAKES ¾ CUP**

PREP TIME: 5 minutes
COOK TIME: None

`30` `V`

1 cup tightly packed fresh basil leaves

½ teaspoon salt

3 tablespoons pine nuts or walnuts

1 to 2 tablespoons water

3 tablespoons extra-virgin olive oil

1. In a blender or food processor (we prefer a blender because we like ours super finely chopped), blend the basil, salt, pine nuts, and water. Keep the blender running while you stream the olive oil in.

2. Transfer to a mason jar or other container with a tightly fitting lid, and store refrigerated for up to 7 days or freeze.

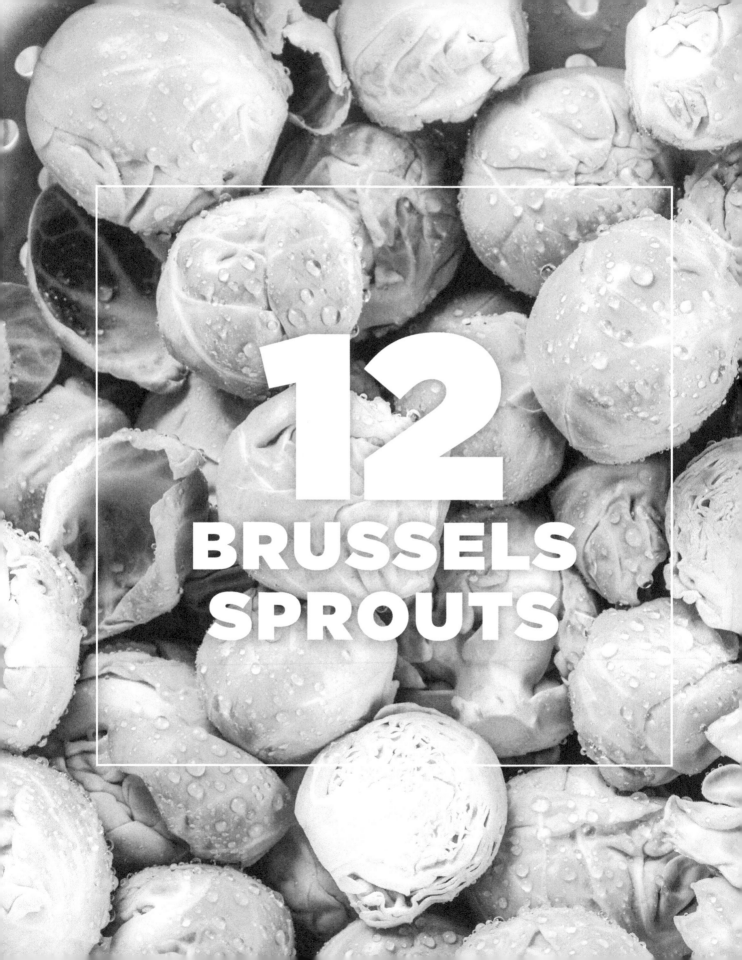

12
BRUSSELS
SPROUTS

Brussels sprouts are my favorite vegetable by far. I love the layered effect of the leaves, plus the fact that you can get them super crispy. They're delicious fried in some butter or ghee or roasted, but that's hardly an exhaustive list of their applications. When thinly sliced, they're surprisingly good in salads, and shredded Brussels sprouts are great when tossed into soups, stir-fries, and even fritters.

I love picking up a 1-pound package of them at the store every week, and even though I usually just roast or pan-fry them, it's always nice to have options, especially since you can do so much with this wonderful little vegetable.

BACON BRUSSELS SPROUTS

Any time I go to a new restaurant and there are Brussels sprouts on the menu, I make sure to order them—they're my favorite vegetable, and I really enjoy encountering new flavor combinations. One of the best I've ever had is the Red Hot Brussels Sprouts from Butcher and the Boar in Minneapolis (a very Paleo-friendly restaurant, if you're ever in the area). The recipe below makes for a great "base Brussels sprout"; it will give you a crunchy and full-flavored Brussels sprout each and every time. **SERVES 2**

PREP TIME: 5 minutes
COOK TIME: 20 minutes

2 slices bacon

2 cups Brussels sprouts, halved

½ to 1 teaspoon salt

¼ teaspoon freshly ground black pepper

1. In a large skillet over medium-high heat, cook the bacon until crispy, about 5 minutes. Transfer the cooked bacon from the skillet to a paper towel–lined plate to drain.

2. Add the Brussels sprouts to the fat in the pan, and cook until golden-brown and crispy, about 15 minutes, stirring occasionally to prevent burning. While the Brussels sprouts cook, cut the bacon into bite-size pieces.

3. Season the Brussels sprouts with salt and pepper, and serve them hot, topped with the chopped bacon.

VARIATION 1 **ASIAN BRUSSELS SPROUTS:** Skip the bacon and sauté the sprouts in a bit of sesame oil for an Asian flavor.

VARIATION 2 **BREAKFAST BRUSSELS SPROUTS:** Top with two fried eggs to create a delicious breakfast—drizzle some olive oil into a hot skillet, and crack the eggs gently into it. Cook on one side until the whites are no longer runny, and then carefully flip and cook for a minute or two on the other side, depending on how done you want the yolks.

PREP TIP: Brussels sprouts keep well in the fridge, so go ahead and slice them as soon as you get them home from the grocery store so they're ready to go anytime.

SHAVED BRUSSELS SPROUT SALAD WITH APPLE CIDER VINAIGRETTE

I don't know why, but I hardly ever do anything with raw Brussels sprouts. This quick and easy dish is what I make when I remember that they're great raw, too. The combination of apple cider and honey with the tender Brussels sprout leaves makes this a perfect salad for spring or fall . . . or summer . . . okay, winter too. **SERVES 4**

PREP TIME: 15 minutes
COOK TIME: None

30 **DF**

1 pound Brussels sprouts

1 small to medium red onion, finely sliced

1 cup chopped almonds

½ cup dried cranberries

1 tablespoon Dijon mustard

2 teaspoons honey

1 garlic clove, minced

3 to 4 tablespoons apple cider vinegar

½ cup extra-virgin olive oil

1. Use a mandolin to very carefully slice the Brussels sprouts. If you have a few extra minutes, you could do this with a knife, or you can quickly pulse them in a food processor or blender. Throw them in a serving bowl with the red onion, almonds, and cranberries.

2. In a separate small bowl, whisk to combine the Dijon mustard, honey, garlic, and apple cider vinegar. Whisk continuously while streaming the olive oil into the bowl.

3. Drizzle a few tablespoons of dressing over the salad, and toss well. Add a little more if you like it more heavily dressed, and serve.

VARIATION 1 **BACON-BRUSSELS SPROUT SALAD WITH GREEN PEAS:** Add ¼ cup raw green peas and ¼ cup sliced sugar snap peas to the salad.

VARIATION 2 **SHAVED BRUSSELS SPROUT SALAD WITH BALSAMIC VINAIGRETTE:** Use the Balsamic Vinaigrette (page 89) instead of making the apple cider vinaigrette for a strong but sweet flavor.

PALEO PAIR: Serve as a side with Prosciutto-Wrapped Pork Tenderloin (page 73).

BRUSSELS SPROUT HASH

This hash makes a wonderful side dish or an amazing breakfast, either on its own or with the addition of eggs. I love how crispy the sprouts can get, and when paired with the spicy sausage, this dish is enormously satisfying. **SERVES 4**

PREP TIME: 10 minutes
COOK TIME: 20 minutes

30 **DF** **NF**

2 teaspoons extra-virgin olive oil

½ onion, diced

1 or 2 garlic cloves, minced

1 pound spicy Italian sausage

1 pound Brussels sprouts, shredded

Salt

Freshly ground black pepper

1. In a large sauté pan over medium heat, heat the olive oil. Sauté the onion until slightly translucent, about 5 minutes.

2. Add the garlic, and stir. Add the sausage, and break it up with a wooden spoon. Cook until no longer pink, about 10 minutes.

3. Move the sausage to one side of the pan, and add the Brussels sprouts. Stir them around so they get coated in some of the sausage fat, and then slowly incorporate everything in the pan. Raise the heat to medium-high, and cook until some of the pieces start to get crispy, about another 5 minutes.

4. Season with salt and pepper, remove from the heat, and serve.

VARIATION 1 **BRUSSELS SPROUT HASH WITH PANCETTA:** Substitute the sausage for ½ pound diced pancetta, and follow the recipe as written. Using pancetta instead of hot Italian sausage takes this from somewhat spicy to a lip-smacking, fattier dish.

VARIATION 2 **BREAKFAST BRUSSELS SPROUT HASH:** Serve topped with 1 or 2 fried eggs for a hearty breakfast—drizzle some olive oil into a hot skillet, and crack the eggs gently into it. Cook on one side until the whites are no longer runny, and then carefully flip and cook for a minute or two on the other side, depending on how done you want the yolks.

PREP TIP: Chop the veggies the night before, and cook everything quickly the morning you plan to serve this dish.

SPICY ROASTED BRUSSELS SPROUTS

This is my version of the Red Hot Brussels Sprouts I mentioned in the Bacon Brussels Sprouts recipe (page 178). It's probably my favorite way to eat Brussels sprouts, and they make a great side dish for any number of entrées or just as a spicy snack. You can totally throw them back in the oven or even pan-fry to reheat, but they won't be quite as good, which is why I make these in smaller batches. **SERVES 4**

PREP TIME: 5 minutes
COOK TIME: 40 minutes

NF

10 ounces Brussels sprouts, halved

½ cup Buffalo Sauce (page 46)

Salt

Freshly ground black pepper

1. Preheat the oven to 400°F.

2. In a large bowl, toss the Brussels sprouts in the Buffalo Sauce, and season with salt and pepper.

3. Spread the Brussels sprouts out on a pan, roast for 35 to 40 minutes, or until crispy, and serve.

VARIATION 1 **BALSAMIC-ROASTED BRUSSELS SPROUTS:** Toss the sprouts with 2 tablespoons extra-virgin olive oil and 3 tablespoons balsamic vinegar. Continue with the recipe as written, but omit the Buffalo Sauce.

VARIATION 2 **GARLIC-ROASTED BRUSSELS SPROUTS:** Toss the sprouts with 3 tablespoons melted butter and 2 to 3 minced garlic cloves. Continue with the recipe as written, but omit the Buffalo Sauce.

PALEO PAIR: Serve these as a side with Burger Bowls (page 51).

ROASTED BRUSSELS SPROUT SKEWERS

These Brussels sprout skewers are a great party vegetable because you can make them ahead of time and then roast (or even grill them, if you're cooking out) right before serving the rest of the food. They do take 30 to 40 minutes to cook, so keep that in mind if you're entertaining. **SERVES 4 TO 6**

PREP TIME: 15 minutes
COOK TIME: 40 minutes

NF **V**

1 pound Brussels sprouts

1 large red onion, quartered, layers separated

1 large yellow squash (or zucchini), quartered lengthwise and chopped

¼ cup extra-virgin olive oil

Salt

Freshly ground black pepper

1. Preheat the oven to 400°F.

2. Carefully skewer a few Brussels sprouts, one layer of onion, and a piece of squash. Repeat until the skewer is full. Place on a roasting pan. Repeat until the vegetables are used up.

3. Brush each skewer with olive oil, and season with salt and pepper. Roast for 30 to 40 minutes, or until the onions are tender and the Brussels sprouts are slightly browned, and serve.

VARIATION 1 **BBQ-ROASTED BRUSSELS SPROUT SKEWERS:** Brush the skewers with BBQ Sauce (page 131).

VARIATION 2 **SWEET POTATO–BRUSSELS SPROUT SKEWERS:** Swap the squash for peeled, diced sweet potato to get some healthy beta-carotene into your system.

PREP TIP: Skewer and marinate the vegetables ahead of time, and pop them in the oven (or onto the grill) about an hour before you want to serve.

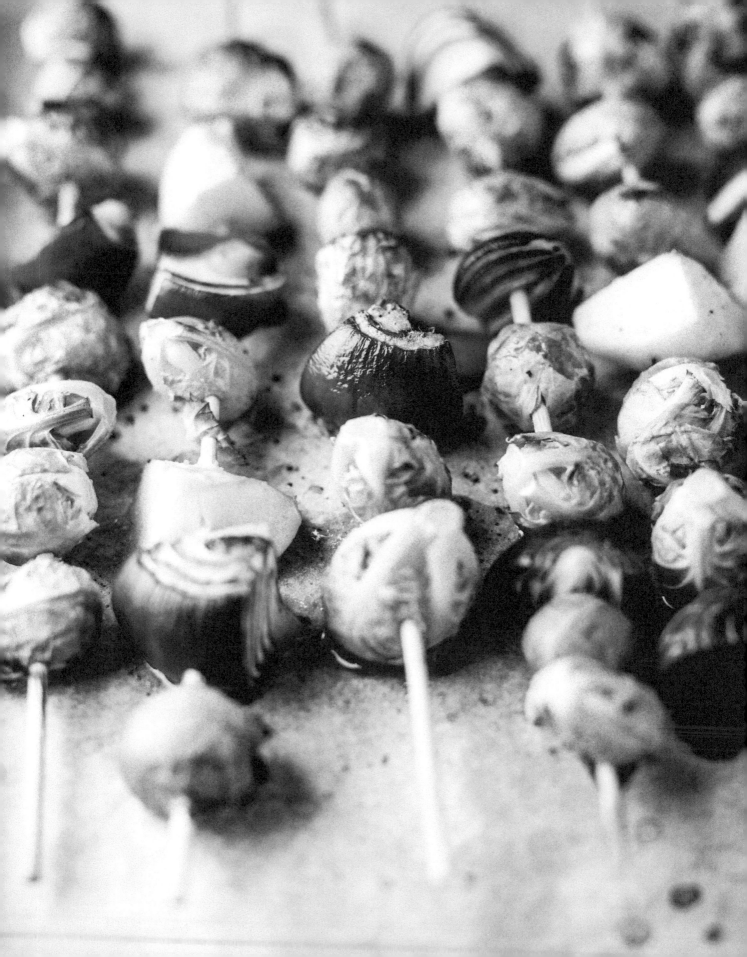

STUFFED BRUSSELS SPROUTS

I think Brussels sprouts are the perfect vegetable for entertaining—you can do so much with them, and you don't need a ton of ingredients to make them delicious. These little stuffed Brussels sprouts make a fantastic appetizer or side dish, and while they're a little labor intensive, they're well worth it. **SERVES 4**

PREP TIME: 20 minutes
COOK TIME: 25 minutes

DF **NF**

1 pound Brussels sprouts, halved

5 to 6 ounces pancetta, finely chopped

1 shallot, minced

1 garlic clove, minced

Freshly ground black pepper

1. Preheat the oven to 400°F.

2. With a small spoon (or your fingers), remove the inside of each Brussels sprout, leaving a thin shell of 1 or 2 layers. Set the two parts aside separately.

3. In a large skillet over medium heat, sauté the pancetta, shallot, and garlic for about 5 minutes (the pancetta will release some fat, so you don't really need any additional oil). Chop the reserved inside parts of the Brussels sprouts, add to the pan, and cook for 5 to 6 minutes more. Remove from the heat, season with pepper, and carefully spoon the mixture into the Brussels sprout shells.

4. Place the stuffed Brussels sprouts on a baking sheet, cook in the oven for 10 to 15 minutes, until tender, and serve.

VARIATION 1 **SAUSAGE-STUFFED BRUSSELS SPROUTS:** For a livelier version, swap the pancetta for hot Italian sausage (the cook time should be about the same).

VARIATION 2 **DATE-STUFFED BRUSSELS SPROUTS:** For a sweeter and vegetarian twist on this dish, chop up ½ cup pitted dates and sauté with onion and garlic in place of the pancetta.

PALEO PAIR: Serve with Beef Tenderloin (page 56).

BRUSSELS SPROUT SOUP WITH SAUSAGE

When I think of making soup, Brussels sprouts don't usually come to mind, but this soup with sausage and lots of Brussels sprouts is super delicious and satisfying. It reminds me of winter weekends when I usually spend a lot of time cooking at home. It's packed with vegetables and meat, so if you have a friend or family member who isn't really into soup (like my husband), you might be able to impress them with this one. **SERVES 4**

PREP TIME: 10 minutes
COOK TIME: 50 minutes

1 pound spicy Italian sausage

2 garlic cloves, minced

1 small onion, diced

1 pound Brussels sprouts, halved

Salt

Freshly ground black pepper

4 to 6 cups beef broth

2 dried bay leaves

1. In a large saucepan over medium-high heat, cook the sausage until it is no longer pink, 5 to 7 minutes. Add the garlic and onion, and sauté with the meat for about 5 minutes more.

2. Add the Brussels sprouts, and continue to sauté for another 5 to 7 minutes, or until they start to brown a bit. Season with salt and pepper, and pour the broth into the pot along with the bay leaves. Bring to a boil, reduce the heat to low, and simmer for at least 30 minutes.

3. Remove the bay leaves and serve.

VARIATION 1 **BRUSSELS SPROUT SOUP WITH SAUSAGE AND SWEET POTATOES:** Add 2 peeled and diced sweet potatoes to the pot 10 to 15 minutes before the Brussels sprouts.

VARIATION 2 **BRUSSELS SPROUT SOUP WITH PANCETTA:** Swap the sausage for 1 pound diced pancetta or thick-cut bacon for a milder version of this soup.

PALEO PAIR: Serve with Kale Salad with Onion and Avocado (page 128) for a nice weekend lunch.

BRUSSELS SPROUT FRITTERS

These fritters are kind of a combination of Broccoli Bites (page 143) and Zucchini-Spinach Fritters (page 153), except using Brussels sprouts instead. These are great on their own, drizzled with a little Ranch Dressing (page 75), or even stacked on top of a salad. **SERVES 4**

PREP TIME: 15 minutes
COOK TIME: 20 minutes

1 pound Brussels sprouts, shredded or thinly sliced with a mandolin

2 garlic cloves, minced

¼ onion, grated

3 eggs, lightly whisked, plus 1 more if needed

¼ cup almond flour, plus more if needed

Salt

Freshly ground black pepper

2 tablespoons grass-fed butter or ghee

1. In a large bowl, mix to combine the Brussels sprouts, garlic, onion, eggs, and almond flour. Season with salt and pepper. The mixture should be wet but not runny, and you should be able to form little palm-size balls out of it with your hands—if it's too runny, add a little extra almond flour; if it's too dry, add another egg or a splash of water.

2. In a large sauté pan over medium-high heat, melt the butter. Working in batches so you don't crowd the pan, carefully drop the fritter balls into the hot pan. Press them down with a spatula so they become more of a patty. Cook for 3 minutes on each side, until tender and lightly browned, and serve.

VARIATION 1 **BRUSSELS SPROUT–ARTICHOKE FRITTERS:** Add ½ can artichoke hearts (very well drained) to the batter, and cook as directed.

VARIATION 2 **BRUSSELS SPROUT FRITTER EGGS BENEDICT:** Make poached eggs and hollandaise according to the recipe on page 25, and then use these Brussels Sprout Fritters as the English muffin bases instead of mushrooms.

PREP TIP: Make these ahead of time and keep warm in the oven (200°F or under) for up to an hour, or refrigerate and reheat in the microwave.

GINGER-GARLIC BRUSSELS SPROUT STIR-FRY

This recipe combines my two favorite things: sautéed Brussels sprouts and Asian flavors. You could make these in the oven, but I prefer pan-frying them with lots of ghee—I've found that to be the best way to get them extra crispy. **SERVES 4**

PREP TIME: 10 minutes
COOK TIME: 20 minutes

30 **NF**

2 heaping tablespoons ghee

½ red onion, thinly sliced

2 or 3 garlic cloves, minced

1 or 2 teaspoons grated fresh ginger

1 pound Brussels sprouts, trimmed and quartered

1 to 2 teaspoons sesame oil

1 tablespoon sesame seeds, for garnish

1. In a large sauté pan over medium heat, melt the ghee. Add the onion, garlic, and ginger, and sauté, stirring, until fragrant, about 2 minutes.

2. Add the Brussels sprouts, and turn the heat up to medium-high. Stir the Brussels sprouts so that all sides are covered with ghee, and then leave them to caramelize on one side.

3. Mix the sprouts around so the other sides make contact with the hot pan. Continue to cook until most of the sides are browned and starting to get crispy, about 15 minutes in total.

4. Remove from the heat, and drizzle with the sesame oil. Stir one more time, garnish with the sesame seeds, and serve.

VARIATION 1 **SPICY STIR-FRIED BRUSSELS SPROUTS:** Add 1 to 2 teaspoons hot chili oil or chili paste to the sprouts while they're cooking.

VARIATION 2 **CILANTRO-LIME BRUSSELS SPROUTS:** Follow the recipe as written, and finish with the juice of ½ lime and 3 tablespoons of chopped fresh cilantro as a garnish.

PALEO PAIR: Serve these sprouts as a side dish with Asian Chicken Legs (page 46).

ASIAN BRUSSELS SPROUT SALAD

This refreshing salad is a great option if you're craving Asian food but don't want to order takeout. The hot, tangy, gingery dressing goes wonderfully with the sprouts and mandarin oranges, but since it's a salad, it makes a lovely side dish or even a light lunch or dinner. It's a wonderful Asian-inspired option that's packed with veggies and perfectly suited for the warmer months. **SERVES 4**

PREP TIME: 15 minutes
COOK TIME: None

1 pound Brussels sprouts, shredded or sliced finely

½ cup sliced scallions

1 (14-ounce) can mandarin oranges in water, drained

1 tablespoon chili garlic paste

½ teaspoon crushed fresh ginger

3 to 4 tablespoons apple cider vinegar

¼ cup extra-virgin olive oil

¼ cup sesame oil

¼ cup sesame seeds

1. In a large bowl, stir to combine the Brussels sprouts, scallions, and mandarin oranges.

2. In a small bowl, whisk to combine the chili garlic paste, ginger, and apple cider vinegar. Whisk continuously while streaming the olive oil and sesame oil into the bowl.

3. Drizzle a few tablespoons of dressing over the salad, and mix well. Add a little more if you like it more heavily dressed. Garnish with the sesame seeds and serve.

VARIATION 1 **ASIAN BRUSSELS SPROUT SALAD WITH SHRIMP:** Add ½ pound grilled or Blackened Shrimp (page 93) to the salad for some extra protein.

VARIATION 2 **SPICY ASIAN BRUSSELS SPROUT SALAD:** Add ¼ to ½ teaspoon red pepper flakes to really give this salad some heat.

PREP TIP: Slice a big bag of Brussels sprouts ahead of time so they're ready to be thrown into any salad at any time.

PANTRY BASIC: CHIMICHURRI

Chimichurri is fabulous on a big juicy flank steak, but it's also fantastic on eggs. If you're a fan of garlic and fresh green herbs, you're going to love it—and it's really good on almost everything, not just steak and eggs. Make it before you start cooking, and give it 20 to 30 minutes to marinate before serving, if you have the time. If you refrigerate any leftovers, make sure to take it out of the refrigerator in plenty of time to let it come back to room temperature, because it will thicken up when chilled. **MAKES ABOUT 1 CUP**

PREP TIME: 5 minutes, plus 20 minutes to marinate
COOK TIME: None

30 **NF** **V**

½ cup extra-virgin olive oil

1 cup packed fresh parsley

2 tablespoons chopped fresh oregano

¼ cup packed fresh cilantro

⅓ cup red wine vinegar

3 garlic cloves

½ shallot

¼ teaspoon red pepper flakes

Pinch salt

Pinch freshly ground black pepper

1. In a food processor or blender, pulse the olive oil, parsley, oregano, cilantro, red wine vinegar, garlic, shallot, red pepper flakes, salt, and pepper until it reaches the consistency you desire—you can do it super liquid-y or quite rough.

2. Let it stand at room temperature for at least 20 minutes before serving.

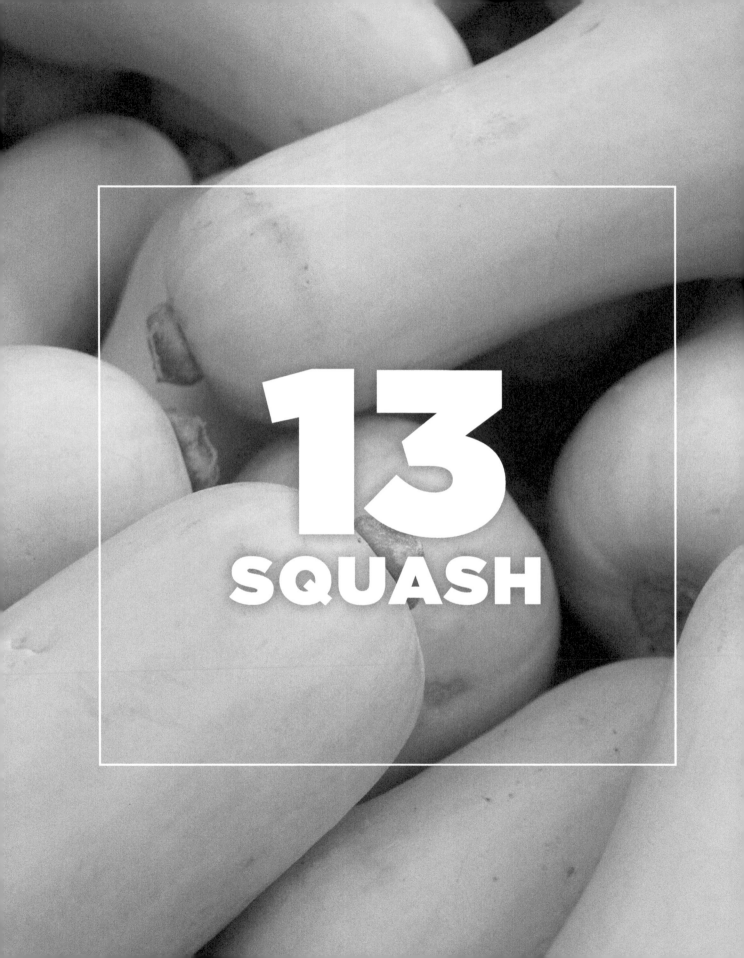

13
SQUASH

This chapter contains a good mix of summer squash (zucchini's yellow cousins) and winter squash, which are hard and have seeds (think butternut or acorn squash). The two have very different flavors and cooking methods, so these recipes are pretty varied.

In the following pages, you'll find a few more noodle recipes (it's just too easy with summer squash), some salads, classic sautéed squash, soup, a casserole, chili, and many more variations.

If a recipe in this chapter calls for winter squash, you can use almost any hard, gourd-like squash you like; and if it calls for yellow or summer squash, you can substitute there as well—zucchini will work just fine. Feel free to mix it up and use your favorites!

SPAGHETTI SQUASH WITH MEAT SAUCE

Spaghetti squash has really become a Paleo staple—long before people were spiralizing zucchini and other squash, the humble spaghetti squash was offering up its succulent flesh, which, when roasted and then raked with a fork, releases into thin strands that resemble angel hair pasta. The texture is really close to pasta, too, with a little crunch that's similar to al dente noodles, and when you serve it with meat sauce, you can barely tell the difference. **SERVES 4**

PREP TIME: 10 minutes
COOK TIME: 1 hour, 15 minutes

`DF` `NF`

1 spaghetti squash, halved

2 tablespoons extra-virgin olive oil

½ medium onion, chopped

3 garlic cloves, chopped

1 pound ground beef

1 (28-ounce) can crushed tomatoes

⅓ cup chopped fresh parsley, plus 1 tablespoon for garnish

½ teaspoon dried basil

½ teaspoon dried oregano

Salt

Freshly ground black pepper

1. Preheat the oven to 400°F. On a large baking sheet, place the two spaghetti squash halves cut-side down and roast for 1 hour.

2. While the squash is roasting, in a large skillet over medium heat, heat the olive oil. Sauté the onion and garlic until the onion is slightly translucent, about 5 minutes. Add the ground beef, and break it apart with a wooden spoon. Cook until no longer pink, 7 to 8 minutes.

3. Add the tomatoes, parsley, basil, and oregano, season with salt and pepper, and simmer on low until the squash has finished cooking.

4. Remove the squash from the oven, and let it cool for a couple of minutes. Rake the flesh out with a fork (you may need to wear an oven mitt on your other hand to steady the squash), and put the "noodles" in a serving bowl. Top with the sauce, garnish with the extra parsley, and serve.

`VARIATION 1` **SPAGHETTI SQUASH WITH MEATBALLS:** Instead of sautéing the meat into the sauce, make Meatballs (page 50) and top the squash with them.

`VARIATION 2` **ZUCCHINI NOODLES WITH MEAT SAUCE:** Make the meat sauce as directed in the original recipe, but cook 3 or 4 spiralized zucchini in the sauce for 3 to 4 minutes before serving.

PREP TIP: Make this sauce ahead of time and freeze. You can also roast the squash and remove the flesh ahead of time.

SAUTÉED SQUASH WITH SUN-DRIED TOMATOES

This squash with sun-dried tomatoes is a wonderful side dish for summer. A big batch of it goes perfectly with burgers or hotdogs at a cookout, but it's also a great option for weeknight dinners and will be great with any chicken, beef, pork, or seafood dish you choose. I love the combination of sun-dried tomatoes with sweet and bright squash, and I think you will too. **SERVES 4**

PREP TIME: 5 minutes
COOK TIME: 15 minutes

`30` `NF` `V`

1 tablespoon extra-virgin olive oil

¼ onion, sliced

2 garlic cloves, minced

2 large yellow squash, diced

3 tablespoons sun-dried tomatoes

Salt

Freshly ground black pepper

1. In a large skillet over medium heat, heat the olive oil. Sauté the onion and garlic until the onion is slightly translucent, about 5 minutes.

2. Add the squash, and stir. Cook for another 5 minutes.

3. Add the sun-dried tomatoes, and sauté for another 2 to 3 minutes.

4. Season with salt and pepper, and serve.

`VARIATION 1` **SAUTÉED SQUASH WITH SUN-DRIED TOMATO AND BASIL PESTO:** Add 2 to 3 tablespoons Pesto (page 175) to the pan with the sun-dried tomatoes, and sauté for 3 to 5 minutes before serving. Garnish with 1 tablespoon chopped fresh basil.

`VARIATION 2` **SAUTÉED ZUCCHINI WITH ROASTED RED PEPPERS:** Substitute zucchini for the yellow squash and 3 or 4 tablespoons chopped roasted red peppers for the sun-dried tomatoes, and enjoy the smoky sweetness.

PALEO PAIR: Serve alongside Green Shrimp or Green Chicken (page 100).

SQUASH NOODLES IN WALNUT-SAGE BUTTER

This is a super easy and really luxurious recipe. The combination of fresh sage and walnuts in a simple butter sauce is a winner. **SERVES 4**

PREP TIME: 10 minutes
COOK TIME: 10 minutes

30

4 tablespoons grass-fed butter

1 small shallot, minced

½ cup chopped walnuts

⅓ cup chopped fresh sage leaves, plus a little extra for garnish

4 large yellow squash, spiralized

Salt

Freshly ground black pepper

1. In a large skillet over medium heat, melt the butter. Sauté the shallot until slightly translucent, about 5 minutes. Add the walnuts and sage, and give it a good stir. Cook for another 2 to 3 minutes, or until the walnuts get a bit toasted.

2. Add the squash noodles to the pan, and sauté until fork-tender, just 2 to 3 minutes more.

3. Season with salt and pepper and serve.

VARIATION 1 **SQUASH NOODLES WITH PESTO:** Skip the walnut-sage butter, and sauté the squash noodles in 2 teaspoons olive oil. Toss with 4 to 5 tablespoons Pesto (page 175).

VARIATION 2 **SQUASH NOODLES WITH MEAT SAUCE:** Sauté 1 pound ground beef and 1 (14-ounce) can diced tomatoes in a large pan until the meat is no longer pink, 7 to 8 minutes. Season with salt and pepper, and add the squash noodles. Cook for another 2 to 3 minutes and serve.

PALEO PAIR: Serve these squash noodles in walnut-sage butter with a side of Perfect Sautéed Mushrooms (page 207) for a light lunch.

SQUASH BISQUE

Thick, creamy butternut squash soup is incredibly comforting and perfect on a chilly fall day, although you could definitely lighten it up and serve it any time of year. Make a big batch of this the next time you find a butternut squash at the market—you'll be glad you did. **SERVES 6 TO 8**

PREP TIME: 10 minutes
COOK TIME: 40 minutes
TOTAL TIME: 55 minutes

NF

3 tablespoons grass-fed butter

1 onion, diced

3 garlic cloves, minced

¼ teaspoon dried thyme

¼ teaspoon red pepper flakes (less if you prefer it milder)

1 large butternut squash, peeled and diced

4 cups chicken broth

1 (13.5-ounce) can full-fat coconut milk

Salt

Freshly ground black pepper

1. In a large saucepan over medium heat, melt the butter. Sauté the onion and garlic until the onion is slightly translucent, about 5 minutes. Add the thyme and red pepper flakes. Stir again and add the squash, quickly sautéing for about 3 minutes.

2. Pour the chicken broth in, and bring to a boil. Reduce the heat to low, and simmer for 20 to 30 minutes. Add the coconut milk, and stir until well incorporated. Remove from the heat.

3. Allow the soup to cool slightly for about 5 minutes, and then carefully blend it, either with an immersion blender or in a regular blender (pour it in and blend it in batches, but don't overfill the blender, and hold a clean dishtowel over the lid while you're blending; hot soup can be volatile).

4. Taste, season with salt and pepper, and serve.

VARIATION 1 **CURRIED SQUASH BISQUE:** Add 1½ tablespoons curry powder to the pan when you add the thyme and red pepper flakes.

VARIATION 2 **CARROT-SQUASH BISQUE:** Add 3 or 4 peeled and chopped carrots to the pan when you add the squash.

PALEO PAIR: Serve this soup with a big side of Kale Salad with Onion and Avocado (page 128).

ROASTED SQUASH WITH CINNAMON

Roasted squash has a lovely sweet quality to it, so it only makes sense to accent that with a drizzle of maple syrup and some cinnamon. This recipe is wonderful around Thanksgiving, maybe with roasted turkey or a ham, but it's great anytime as a twist on your usual savory vegetables. You can use any firm squash you like, but my favorite for this recipe is butternut. **SERVES 4**

PREP TIME: 10 minutes
COOK TIME: 30 minutes

1 large butternut squash, peeled and sliced lengthwise into 1-inch pieces

2 tablespoons extra-virgin olive oil

1 tablespoon maple syrup

2 teaspoons ground cinnamon

1. Preheat the oven to 400°F.

2. In a large bowl, toss the butternut squash with the olive oil and maple syrup.

3. Transfer to a baking sheet, and sprinkle with the cinnamon. Bake for 25 to 30 minutes, or until fork-tender, and serve.

VARIATION 1 **PLAIN ROASTED SQUASH:** Skip the cinnamon and maple syrup, and season the butternut squash with olive oil, salt, and pepper. Roast at 400°F for 25 to 30 minutes.

VARIATION 2 **ROSEMARY-GARLIC ROASTED SQUASH:** Toss the squash in olive oil with 3 cloves minced garlic, 2 or 3 chopped rosemary sprigs, and ¼ cup pumpkin seeds. Season with salt and pepper, and roast according to the original recipe.

PREP TIP: Peel and dice hard squashes as soon as you get them home from the grocery store if you know you'll be cooking them within 3 or 4 days. The chopping is by far the most difficult part of any squash recipe, so doing it ahead of time will be worth it later.

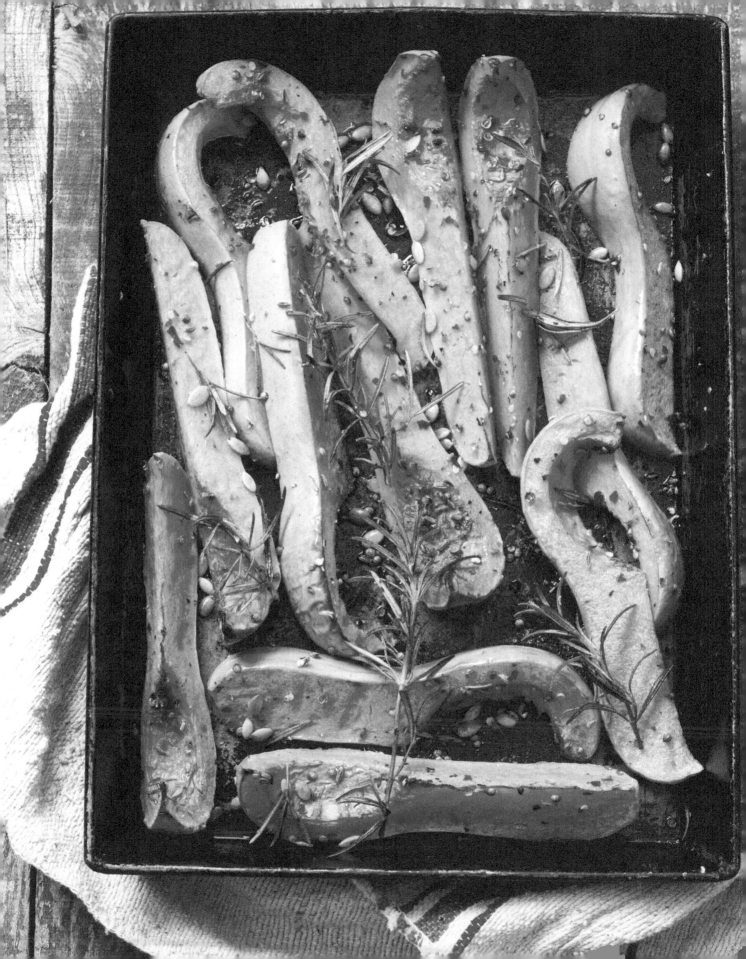

SQUASH CASSEROLE

Summer squash is so versatile but for some reason never got any of the hype that zucchini did, and I'm not sure why—you can still make it into noodles, cut it up and have it raw with Beet Hummus (page 170) or Ranch Dressing (page 75), just sauté it in some garlic for a delicious and easy vegetable option, or bake it in this delicious casserole. I love its mild flavor and easy-to-work-with texture. **SERVES 4**

PREP TIME: 15 minutes
COOK TIME: 50 minutes

½ tablespoon grass-fed butter, plus more for greasing

1 onion, sliced

2 garlic cloves, minced

4 eggs, whisked

1 tablespoon extra-virgin olive oil

2 tablespoons canned full-fat coconut milk

5 tablespoons almond flour, divided

Salt

Freshly ground black pepper

4 or 5 yellow squash, cut into thin coins

2 to 3 tablespoons sliced scallion, for garnish

1. Preheat the oven to 350°F.

2. In a medium sauté pan over medium heat, melt the butter. Cook the onion and garlic until the onion is slightly translucent, about 5 minutes.

3. In a large bowl, mix together the eggs, olive oil, coconut milk, and 2½ tablespoons of almond flour. Season the mixture with salt and pepper.

4. Add the squash to the mixture in batches (like you're battering it). Butter an 8-by-12-inch baking dish, and layer the squash into it. Add some of the cooked onions and garlic, and repeat. Once you've finished battering the squash and it's all in the baking dish, pour the remaining egg mixture over the top of the squash. Season again with a little more salt and pepper, then sprinkle the remaining 2½ tablespoons of almond flour on top and bake for 45 minutes, until lightly browned.

5. Serve hot, garnished with the scallions.

VARIATION 1 **SQUASH AND CARROT CASSEROLE:** Add 1 cup grated carrots to the baking dish with the onion and garlic.

VARIATION 2 **SQUASH MEDLEY CASSEROLE:** Make this casserole with 2 yellow squash and 2 zucchini squash for a bit more color.

PALEO PAIR: I love this as a side dish with Roasted Lemon Chicken (page 40).

BUTTERNUT SQUASH CHILI

This chili is really similar to the Chicken Chili (page 42), but I swapped the meat for diced squash to make it vegetarian. There's also vegetable broth instead of chicken broth, but if you wanted to make squash chili and use chicken broth (or even use beef broth for more flavor), you could do that. Chili is a wonderful dish to make in the fall, and this butternut squash version is a seasonal treat that I think you're really going to love. **SERVES 4 TO 6**

PREP TIME: 20 minutes
COOK TIME: 2 hours, 30 minutes

2 tablespoons extra-virgin olive oil

1 large onion, diced

2 or 3 garlic cloves, chopped

1 medium red bell pepper, chopped

1 medium yellow bell pepper, chopped

1 large butternut squash, peeled and diced

1 (28-ounce) can crushed tomatoes

1 tablespoon chili powder

1½ teaspoons red pepper flakes

1 teaspoon ground cumin

1 teaspoon ground paprika

¾ teaspoon ground coriander

¾ teaspoon dried mustard

½ teaspoon ground allspice

½ teaspoon dried oregano

2 cups vegetable broth, divided

1½ teaspoons ground cayenne pepper (more or less depending on your heat preference)

½ cup apple cider vinegar

2 to 3 tablespoons sliced scallions, for garnish

1. In a large cast iron pot over medium heat, heat the olive oil. Sauté the onion, garlic, and red and yellow bell peppers until they have cooked down a bit, about 5 minutes.

2. Add the diced squash, and sauté for another 10 to 15 minutes.

3. Once the squash is approaching fork-tenderness, add the tomatoes. Give it a good stir, and add the chili powder, red pepper flakes, cumin, paprika, coriander, mustard, allspice, and oregano.

4. Add 1 cup of broth to the pot, raise the heat to medium-high, and bring the chili to a low boil. Reduce the heat to simmer, and cook for at least 2 hours. Stir in the remaining 1 cup of broth in increments when the chili starts getting thick.

5. About 20 minutes before serving, add the cayenne by the ½ teaspoon (so you can adjust the level of heat to your preference), and stir in the apple cider vinegar. Garnish with the scallions.

VARIATION 1 **MEATY CHILI:** Use turkey or beef instead of (or in addition to) the squash for a heartier texture and flavor.

VARIATION 2 **MUSHROOM AND SQUASH CHILI:** Add 10 ounces chopped white button mushrooms to the chili when you add the squash.

PALEO PAIR: Serve with a side of Plain Cauliflower Rice (page 116).

SQUASH RIBBON SALAD WITH APPLES AND WALNUTS

This is a really interesting salad to eat for lunch, with lots of texture and flavor going on. The combination of kale, apples, and squash already makes it feel pretty autumnal. Add some walnuts for crunch and a splash of apple cider vinegar and you've got a really delicious fall or winter salad. **SERVES 2**

PREP TIME: 15 minutes
COOK TIME: None

1 tablespoon minced shallot

1 to 2 tablespoons honey

¼ cup apple cider vinegar

½ cup extra-virgin olive oil

1½ to 2 cups kale, stemmed

1 apple, cored and sliced

1 yellow squash, spiralized or cut into thin ribbons with a vegetable peeler

½ cup walnuts

Salt

Freshly ground black pepper

1. In a small bowl, mix to combine the shallot with the honey, apple cider vinegar, and olive oil. In a large serving bowl, pour the dressing over the kale and mix in well with your hands or a wooden spoon (3 to 5 minutes of mixing will make the kale leaves much softer and easier to eat).

2. Add the apple, squash noodles, and walnuts, and give it a good toss. Season with salt and pepper, and serve.

VARIATION 1 **SQUASH RIBBON SALAD WITH POMEGRANATE:** Add ¼ to ½ cup pomegranate seeds to the salad for some extra color and juiciness.

VARIATION 2 **MUSHROOM-KALE SALAD:** Instead of apples, squash, and walnuts, top this salad with a few tablespoons of marinated mushrooms (like the Button Mushroom Ceviche on page 206).

PREP TIP: Massaging the raw kale with the dressing takes a few minutes but is well worth the effort as the leaves become tender and easier to eat. If you know you're going to be short on time later in the day, try to fit in this step earlier so you'll be ready to just assemble the salad and enjoy.

SQUASH BREAKFAST SKILLET

This recipe is a squash-y take on Baked Eggs in Tomato Sauce (page 22). They're still baked in a tomato sauce, but lots of fresh summer squash is added to up the vegetable count. Squash and tomatoes go so well together, and with baked eggs, this one-pot breakfast dish is what dreams are made of. Topped with fresh basil, you've got yourself a really beautiful summer breakfast. **SERVES 4 TO 6**

PREP TIME: 10 minutes
COOK TIME: 25 minutes

DF **NF**

4 summer squash of your choice

1 tablespoon extra-virgin olive oil

1 small onion, chopped

2 garlic cloves, minced

1 (16-ounce) can diced tomatoes, drained

1 teaspoon ground paprika

½ to 1 teaspoon red pepper flakes

Salt

Freshly ground black pepper

6 eggs

Fresh basil, for garnish

1. Preheat the oven to 375°F.

2. Trim and discard the ends of the squash. Grate them, and then use your hands or a clean dishtowel to squeeze out as much water as possible.

3. In an ovenproof skillet over medium heat, heat the olive oil. Sauté the onion and garlic until the onion is slightly translucent, about 5 minutes. Add the squash and tomatoes, and cook for about 10 minutes, or until any liquid in the pan starts to evaporate.

4. Season with the paprika, red pepper flakes, salt, and pepper, and then create 6 wells in the mixture. Crack 1 egg into each well, and transfer to the oven to bake until the whites have set, 7 to 10 minutes.

5. Garnish with the basil, and serve.

VARIATION 1 **SWEET POTATO BREAKFAST SKILLET:** Make the recipe above with 4 sweet potatoes instead of squash—just shred or chop the sweet potatoes into small cubes and cook in the pan for an additional 4 to 5 minutes before baking.

VARIATION 2 **BAKED EGG SQUASH BITES:** Transfer the sautéed onion and squash to a muffin tin, crack an egg on top of each bite, and continue with the recipe as written.

PREP TIP: Shred the squash ahead of time and add it to recipes as you need it.

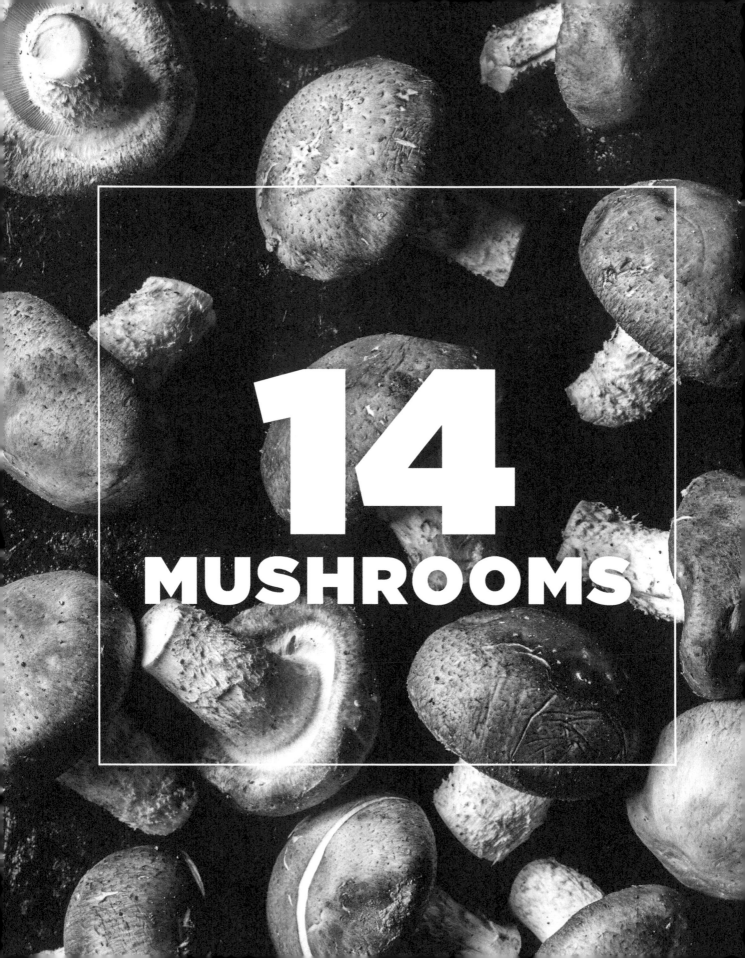

14
MUSHROOMS

I make sautéed mushrooms as a side dish with dinner at least once or twice a week, but lately I've been also using them as a meat substitute. They have great texture and flavor, and if you get big ones like portobellos, you can give them a starring role in a main dish. Vegetarians often use mushrooms as the main ingredient, and I think Paleo eaters can (and should!) do the same from time to time.

Most of the recipes in this chapter call for a specific mushroom (mostly button or baby bella), but if you like one type more than another, you can absolutely substitute. The Marinated Portobello Mushrooms (page 210) might be difficult to make with smaller mushrooms, but if you don't lose them on the grill, they'll still be delicious. I usually buy a 10-ounce prepackaged box of regular white mushrooms every week, but if there are wilder varieties available at the store (shiitake, morels, etc.), I love to mix it up.

STUFFED MUSHROOMS

Stuffed mushrooms are an awesome appetizer. They do require a bit of work to make, but they're always popular. You can stuff them with many different kinds of fillings, but my favorite is a simple mix of crab meat, scallion, and a splash of lemon juice. **SERVES 4**

PREP TIME: 20 minutes
COOK TIME: 15 minutes

DF **NF**

20 to 24 ounces whole mushrooms (white or baby bellas)

12 ounces canned crab

¼ cup fresh basil, chopped, divided

Juice of 1 lemon

Salt

Freshly ground black pepper

1. Preheat the oven to 350°F.

2. Wash the mushrooms (if you don't like to wash them, you can wipe them down with a damp paper towel, although I've found that rinsing them in water doesn't really mess up the texture the way some people think it does) and remove the stems—you can just pop them right off. Spoon out the fibrous underside so the mushrooms are hollow.

3. In a large bowl, mix to combine the crab, most of the basil (reserve 2 tablespoons for garnish), and the lemon juice. Season with salt and pepper, and then spoon some filling into each mushroom cap. Put them on a baking sheet and cook in the oven for 15 minutes.

4. Garnish with the remaining 2 tablespoons of basil and serve.

VARIATION 1 **SHRIMP-STUFFED MUSHROOMS:** Use 12 ounces cooked shrimp instead of crab—make sure to chop it really finely. Follow the rest of the recipe as written.

VARIATION 2 **SAUSAGE-STUFFED MUSHROOMS:** Sauté ¼ onion, chopped, with 2 or 3 cloves minced garlic in 1 tablespoon olive oil for 5 minutes. Add ½ pound spicy Italian sausage, and cook until no longer pink, another 5 minutes. Remove from the heat, cool, and use the mixture to stuff the mushrooms.

PREP TIP: You can chop up the mushroom stems and sauté them quickly before adding them to the filling if you don't want to throw them away. Also, you can assemble these stuffed mushrooms ahead of time and refrigerate or freeze them until ready to bake.

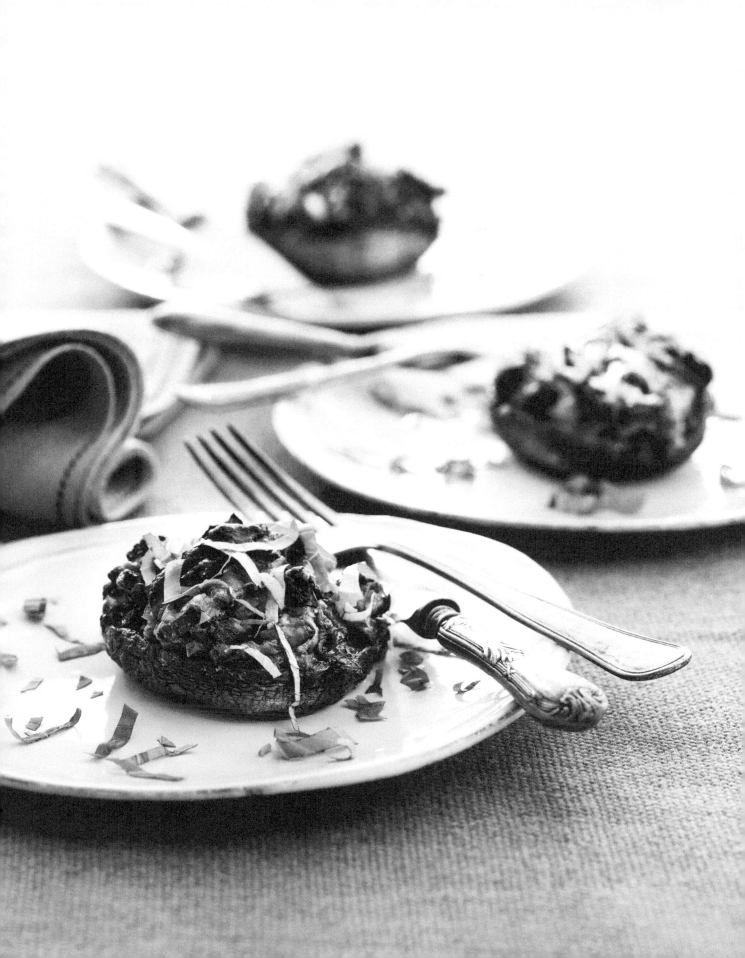

BUTTON MUSHROOM CEVICHE

This recipe was inspired by two completely different things: first, a trip I took to Miami where I ate almost nothing but ceviche for three whole days, and second, those little marinated, almost-pickled mushrooms you sometimes find in olive bars at fancy food markets. Funny how two different memories can bring you to the same place in the here and now. **SERVES 4**

PREP TIME: 10 minutes, plus 30 minutes to marinate
COOK TIME: None

10 ounces small button mushrooms (the smaller the better)

3 or 4 tablespoons extra-virgin olive oil (just under ¼ cup)

Juice of 2 juicy limes

Juice of 1 large lemon

1 large shallot or ½ red onion, thinly sliced

1 garlic clove, minced

Salt

Freshly ground black pepper

Sliced scallions or cilantro, for garnish

1. In a large bowl, combine the mushrooms, olive oil, lime juice, lemon juice, shallot, and garlic, and stir gently. Season with salt and pepper. Marinate in the refrigerator for at least 30 minutes, and up to 3 hours.

2. Taste and season again with salt and pepper, if needed. Garnish with scallions and serve.

VARIATION 1 **SPICY MUSHROOM CEVICHE:** Add ½ fresh jalapeño pepper (seeded and finely chopped) to the marinade.

VARIATION 2 **VEGGIE MUSHROOM CEVICHE:** Add ½ sliced green bell pepper, ½ sliced red bell pepper, and 1 shredded carrot to the mushrooms and marinade.

PREP TIP: You can leave these in the fridge for up to a day, so make them ahead of time if you want to get ahead on your meal or party planning.

PERFECT SAUTÉED MUSHROOMS

I make these at least once a week, as my husband and I both really enjoy them. The secret is butter and pretty high heat, in a skillet that's large enough to have mostly one layer of mushrooms so you aren't steaming them. "Don't crowd the mushrooms," said Julia Child, and that woman knew what she was talking about. **SERVES 4**

PREP TIME: 5 minutes
COOK TIME: 15 minutes

2 or 3 tablespoons grass-fed butter

10 ounces mushrooms, sliced

Salt

Freshly ground black pepper

1. In a large skillet over medium-high heat, melt the butter. Add the mushrooms, and stir them around until all sides are coated with butter. Season with salt and pepper. Cook for about 5 minutes before stirring again, and then cook for another 5 minutes or so.

2. Continue stirring and letting them rest until all sides of the mushrooms are browned and beginning to get crispy.

3. Serve immediately.

VARIATION 1 GARLIC SAUTÉED MUSHROOMS: Add 2 cloves minced garlic to the pan with the butter, and follow the recipe as written.

VARIATION 2 SAUTÉED MUSHROOM MEDLEY: Add more flavor and texture to this dish by using a variety of wild mushrooms like cremini, shiitake, and portobello. Slice the larger ones but leave smaller, more bite-size ones whole.

PALEO PAIR: These are delicious as a side with Roasted Lemon Chicken (page 40), another recipe inspired by Julia Child.

MUSHROOM AND SAUSAGE STUFFING

My mom made this stuffing for our first Paleo Thanksgiving. I remember being really hesitant about it, wondering what in the world Thanksgiving might be like without creamy mashed potatoes and bread stuffing. It may be different, but it's still delicious, and this stuffing does a pretty good job filling in for traditional bread stuffing. **SERVES 6 TO 8**

PREP TIME: 10 minutes
COOK TIME: 45 minutes

NF

4 tablespoons grass-fed butter, divided

4 onions, sliced

1 pound ground pork sausage

4 (10-ounce) packages mushrooms, diced (6 cups)

Salt

Freshly ground black pepper

½ cup white wine or chicken broth

½ teaspoon dried oregano

½ teaspoon dried tarragon

¼ teaspoon red pepper flakes

1. In a large skillet over low heat, melt 2 tablespoons of butter. Sauté the onions for 30 minutes, stirring occasionally. Add the sausage to the skillet, and cook until browned, 5 to 7 minutes.

2. Turn the heat up to medium-high, and add the mushrooms. Season with salt and pepper. Stir well and cook for about 10 minutes, or until the mushrooms begin to brown.

3. Add the wine or chicken broth to the skillet, and deglaze the pan, stirring to scrape up the browned bits from the bottom. Lower the heat to low, and add the remaining 2 tablespoons of butter. Stir well so everything gets incorporated.

4. Add the oregano, tarragon, and red pepper flakes, and stir again before serving.

VARIATION 1 **BAKED SAUSAGE AND MUSHROOM STUFFING:** Prepare the recipe as written, and then transfer everything to an 8-by-12-inch baking dish. Mix ½ cup almond flour with 2 or 3 tablespoons melted butter. Crumble over the stuffing, and broil quickly in the oven (3 to 4 minutes at the most) to toast the topping.

VARIATION 2 **SAUSAGE AND MUSHROOM STUFFING WITH CELERY AND CARROTS:** Sauté 2 chopped celery stalks and 2 or 3 large diced carrots with the onions. Continue with the rest of the recipe as written.

PREP TIP: The onions take a full half hour to cook, so either do them ahead of time or plan to do another kitchen task while those are on the stove.

CREAM OF MUSHROOM SOUP

This mushroom soup is really creamy and really good. I know thick, cheesy soups can be incredibly comforting in the colder months, but this beef broth base (say that five times fast) does the trick with the help of a can of full-fat coconut milk. It all gets blended at the end to get that fantastic, thick consistency, and it's finished with a sprinkle of sliced scallions to brighten it up. **SERVES 4**

PREP TIME: 10 minutes
COOK TIME: 30 minutes

NF

2 tablespoons grass-fed butter

1 large shallot, chopped

3 garlic cloves, chopped

16 ounces mushrooms, roughly chopped

4 cups beef broth

2 dried bay leaves

1 (13.5-ounce) can full-fat coconut milk, refrigerated

Salt

Freshly ground black pepper

2 or 3 tablespoons sliced scallions, for garnish

1. In a large saucepan over medium heat, melt the butter. Sauté the shallot and garlic for 2 minutes. Add the mushrooms, and stir. Raise the heat to medium-high, and cook for about 10 minutes, or until the mushrooms start to brown.

2. Add the broth and bay leaves to the pan, and bring to a low boil. Reduce the heat to low, and simmer for 15 minutes. Add the cream from the top of the can of coconut milk, and season with salt and pepper.

3. Remove from the heat, and carefully purée with an immersion blender (or pour the soup into a blender in batches and purée, holding a clean dishtowel over the lid while blending to prevent potential eruptions).

4. Serve with a pinch of sliced scallions.

VARIATION 1 PALEO CREAM OF MUSHROOM SOUP WITH TRUFFLE OIL: For a really special twist, follow the recipe as written but finish with a tiny drizzle of truffle oil as a garnish. (Truffle oil is pretty expensive but also incredibly potent—even a small bottle will last a long time. It does best without a lot of heat, so add it to dishes once they've finished cooking.)

VARIATION 2 HEARTY MUSHROOM CHOWDER: Chop 2 or 3 celery stalks and 4 or 5 carrots, and add them to the shallot and garlic. Add an extra 5 or 6 ounces mushrooms with the broth and bay leaves in step 2. Skip the blending.

PALEO PAIR: Use this soup as an appetizer course before serving Beef Tenderloin (page 56).

MARINATED PORTOBELLO MUSHROOMS

For some reason, these marinated portobello mushrooms always remind me of my mom, which is funny because I don't think she makes them that often—I guess she did once or twice, and I really remembered them. (It's the same way with lavender—she doesn't even like it much, but I think of her every time I smell it.) Marinated portobello mushrooms make a great vegetarian option for a burger patty, or you can slice them up and add them to salads. **SERVES 4**

PREP TIME: 5 minutes, plus 30 minutes to marinate
COOK TIME: 20 minutes

NF **V**

1 cup extra-virgin olive oil

½ cup balsamic vinegar

1 tablespoon Dijon mustard

2 or 3 garlic cloves, minced

4 large portobello mushroom caps, cleaned and stemmed

Salt

Freshly ground black pepper

1. In a large bowl, mix the olive oil, balsamic vinegar, Dijon mustard, and garlic. Add the portobello mushroom caps to the mixture, and mix well to cover all surfaces. Season with salt and pepper, cover the bowl, and marinate for at least 30 minutes.

2. Remove the mushrooms from the marinade, and cook on a grill, grill pan, or in a regular skillet over medium-high heat for 7 to 10 minutes on each side, until tender, and serve.

VARIATION 1 **ASIAN-MARINATED PORTOBELLO MUSHROOMS:** Marinate the mushrooms in a mixture of ½ cup olive oil, ½ cup sesame oil, and ½ cup apple cider vinegar. Follow the rest of the recipe as written, and garnish with 1 tablespoon sesame seeds.

VARIATION 2 **HERBY GRILLED PORTOBELLO MUSHROOMS:** Use the Green Shrimp marinade (page 100) on your portobello mushrooms. Follow the rest of the recipe as written.

PREP TIP: You can marinate these longer than 30 minutes if you want to get them ready the night before and leave them in the refrigerator until ready to cook.

STEWED MUSHROOMS

For a while I called this "mushroom stew," but it didn't quite feel right. They're definitely comforting and kind of cozy, but really they're stewed mushrooms more than they're mushroom stew. Anyway, I liked the idea of slow-cooking mushrooms in some liquid as opposed to high heat with butter as I usually do. Lots of mushrooms, a little beef broth, and some garlic, finished with a little coconut milk for creaminess . . . and baby, you've got a stew going. (*Arrested Development*, anyone?) **SERVES 4**

PREP TIME: 5 minutes
COOK TIME: 30 minutes

DF **NF**

2 to 4 tablespoons extra-virgin olive oil, divided

¼ onion, diced

2 or 3 garlic cloves, minced

14 ounces mushrooms (sliced baby bellas, shiitake, or whole button)

¼ teaspoon dried oregano

¼ teaspoon dried sage

Salt

Freshly ground black pepper

1 cup beef broth

¼ cup canned full-fat coconut milk

1. In a medium saucepan over medium heat, heat 1 to 2 tablespoons of olive oil. Sauté the onion and garlic until the onion is slightly translucent, about 5 minutes. Add the mushrooms, stir well, and raise the heat to medium-high. Cook for about 10 minutes. Season with the oregano, sage, salt, and pepper.

2. Add the beef broth, and bring to a low boil. Reduce the heat to low, and simmer for 15 minutes, or until some of the liquid has evaporated and reduced to a thicker consistency.

3. Stir in the coconut milk, remove from the heat, and serve.

VARIATION 1 **STEWED MUSHROOM AND LEEKS:** Add some fresh onion flavor to the stew with 1 large sliced leek (only use the white and very light green part). Sauté with the onions, and follow the rest of the recipe as written.

VARIATION 2 **NON-CREAMY STEWED MUSHROOMS:** Brighten this recipe up by skipping the coconut cream and adding a splash of apple cider vinegar to the pan at the end.

PALEO PAIR: Serve these mushrooms as a side with Prosciutto-Wrapped Pork Tenderloin (page 73).

SOUTHERN-STYLE MUSHROOM-SAUSAGE GRAVY

Living in the South but being Paleo means passing on a lot of really delicious Southern food, like chicken and waffles, cheesy grits, and sausage gravy poured over biscuits. This recipe is a Paleo version of sausage gravy, but we've loaded it with mushrooms and have no intention of putting it on a biscuit. **SERVES 4**

PREP TIME: 10 minutes
COOK TIME: 20 minutes

30

1 pound spicy pork sausage

10 ounces mushrooms, diced

3 tablespoons almond flour

½ to ¾ cup almond milk

2 tablespoons grass-fed butter

Salt

Freshly ground black pepper

1. In a large skillet over medium heat, sauté the sausage until is no longer pink, about 10 minutes. Move it all to the edges, and add the mushrooms to the center of the skillet. Raise the heat to medium-high, and brown the mushrooms, 5 to 7 minutes, before stirring the meat and mushrooms together. Sprinkle the almond flour over the mixture to thicken it.

2. Reduce the heat to medium-low, and add the almond milk. Stir well, and add the butter a little at a time, stirring it in until it melts. Season with salt and pepper and serve.

VARIATION 1 **MUSHROOM-SAUSAGE GRAVY AND EGGS:** Scramble 6 eggs (for 4 people), and top with this mushroom-sausage gravy.

VARIATION 2 **MUSHROOM-TURKEY SAUSAGE AND GRAVY:** Use turkey (or chicken sausage) instead of spicy pork sausage for a milder version.

PALEO PAIR: Serve on top of Plain Cauliflower Rice (page 109) for a warm and comforting lunch.

ROASTED MUSHROOM LETTUCE CUPS

I think that, most of the time, Paleo gets a bad rep for being meat-obsessed. I always enjoyed the "more vegetables than a vegetarian" notion, which basically is exactly what it sounds like: If you eat Paleo, you should be striving to eat more vegetables than you imagine a vegetarian would. These roasted mushroom lettuce cups are a great way to do just that. This recipe could just as easily be meat based, but we're going to use mushrooms instead—because sometimes, we should. **SERVES 4**

PREP TIME: 10 minutes
COOK TIME: 30 minutes

NF V

10 ounces baby bella or button mushrooms

2 tablespoons extra-virgin olive oil

1½ teaspoons garlic powder

Salt

Freshly ground black pepper

2 teaspoons sesame oil

1½ teaspoons Asian chili paste or chili oil

4 romaine or butter lettuce leaves, plus a few extra

2 to 3 tablespoons sesame seeds, for garnish

2 to 3 tablespoons chopped fresh cilantro, for garnish

1. Preheat the oven to 450°F.

2. On a large baking sheet, mix the mushrooms with the olive oil and garlic powder, and season with salt and pepper. Roast for 25 to 30 minutes, or until the mushrooms are browned and slightly shrunken. Transfer to a bowl, and toss with the sesame oil and chili paste.

3. Serve the mushrooms on the lettuce leaves, garnished with the sesame seeds and cilantro.

VARIATION 1 **SHIITAKE MUSHROOM LETTUCE CUPS:** Make this recipe with shiitake mushrooms for even more texture and Asian flair.

VARIATION 2 **SPICY PORK-MUSHROOM LETTUCE CUPS:** Go on, add the meat—sauté ½ pound spicy pork sausage while the mushrooms are roasting, and combine them in a large bowl. Top the lettuce leaves with the mixture, and garnish with the sesame seeds and cilantro.

PREP TIP: Make the filling ahead of time and reheat before serving.

GRILLED MUSHROOM SALAD

I had a really awesome salad once with my friend Blair at a restaurant in Charlotte called Luna's Living Kitchen; it was a huge bowl of kale greens topped with the most delicious mushrooms I'd ever eaten. That restaurant is a mostly raw vegan place, so I think they prepared them closer to the Button Mushroom Ceviche (page 206) than this recipe, but it definitely inspired me to start playing with mushroom textures, and also adding them to salads, as here. **SERVES 2**

PREP TIME: 10 minutes
COOK TIME: 5 minutes

30 **NF** **V**

¼ cup balsamic vinegar

½ cup extra-virgin olive oil

1 tablespoon Dijon mustard

1 garlic clove, minced

6 to 8 ounces mushrooms, sliced (shiitake or portobello)

2 to 3 cups arugula greens

½ cup cherry tomatoes, sliced

Salt

Freshly ground black pepper

1. In a large bowl, mix together the vinegar, olive oil, Dijon mustard, and garlic. Add the mushrooms, and stir well to cover all sides with the dressing.

2. Use a slotted spoon to transfer the mushrooms to a large grill pan (or a regular skillet) over medium-high heat, and quickly cook the mushrooms for 3 to 5 minutes.

3. Toss the arugula with the dressing you marinated the mushrooms in, and add the tomatoes. Season with salt and pepper, top with the warm mushrooms, and serve.

VARIATION 1 **SESAME-MUSHROOM SALAD:** Swap the balsamic vinegar for white vinegar and the olive oil for sesame oil. Garnish the salad with 1 tablespoon sesame seeds.

VARIATION 2 **BACON OR PANCETTA MUSHROOM SALAD:** In a skillet over medium-high heat, cook 4 slices bacon (or ½ cup diced pancetta) until crispy, about 5 minutes. Remove from the pan, and sauté the mushrooms in the fat. Break up the cooled bacon into bite-size pieces, and top the salad with the bacon and mushrooms. Make the marinade from the original recipe into a dressing.

PREP TIP: Cook the mushrooms ahead of time, and warm them up in the microwave for 30 seconds before topping the salad with them.

PANTRY BASIC: KETCHUP

I don't use ketchup very often, but when you're eating something that really needs it, it can be difficult to ignore ready-made packets or bottles of ketchup, which are pretty high in added sugar. This Paleo ketchup recipe is a bit on the tart side since it doesn't have any sugar in it, but with a little bit of honey, it does a great job balancing that sweet-tart thing that makes ketchup so delicious. **MAKES ABOUT 1½ CUPS**

PREP TIME: 5 minutes
COOK TIME: None

DF NF

1 (6-ounce) can tomato paste

⅓ cup water

2 tablespoons white vinegar

1 tablespoon honey or maple syrup

¼ teaspoon ground allspice

¼ teaspoon ground cinnamon

¼ teaspoon dried mustard

⅛ teaspoon ground cayenne pepper

Pinch salt

1. In a mason jar or other container with a tightly fitting lid, mix to combine the tomato paste, water, white vinegar, honey, allspice, cinnamon, mustard, cayenne pepper, and salt.

2. Cover and refrigerate for at least 8 hours before serving.

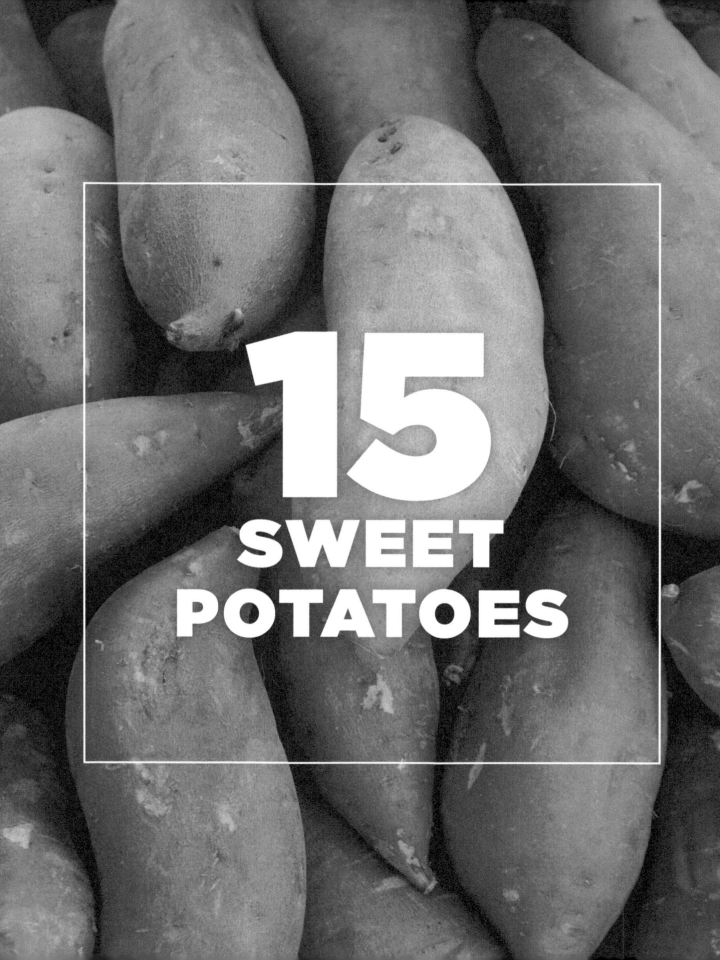

15
SWEET POTATOES

Sweet potatoes are certainly one of the most popular foods you'll see, make, eat, and hear about when you're following the Paleo diet. I was never a huge fan until after I changed the way I eat—for a long time I tried to treat them as a substitute for regular potatoes, and they're just so different in flavor that it didn't work (really, I think the Paleo substitution for white potatoes is cauliflower).

But as soon as I stopped treating sweet potatoes as a replacement for something else, I started really liking them. Sweet Potato Fries (page 218) are always delicious, and here you'll find three variations, but my favorite recipe in this chapter is definitely the Sweet Potato Hash Browns (page 228). All these recipes make great side dishes, and there are even a few entrées as well, like BBQ-Stuffed Sweet Potatoes (page 224) and a Sweet Potato Soup (page 223) that could go either way.

CHILI-LIME SWEET POTATO FRIES

Sweet potato fries are great on their own, but they're even better with a little heat and a fresh squeeze of lime juice. These fries are awesome as a side dish or even just as a snack or appetizer. You can adjust the amount of cayenne pepper depending on how spicy you like them—this recipe calls for ¼ teaspoon, and that's definitely enough for a moderate to high level of spiciness. **SERVES 4**

PREP TIME: 10 minutes
COOK TIME: 20 minutes

2 large sweet potatoes, scrubbed and cut into wedges

2 tablespoons extra-virgin olive oil

¼ teaspoon ground cayenne pepper

Salt

Freshly ground black pepper

Juice of ½ lime

Chimichurri (page 189), for dipping (optional)

1. Preheat the oven to 400°F.

2. Spread the sweet potato wedges out over a large baking sheet. Drizzle with the olive oil and sprinkle with the cayenne. Mix around well with your hands (make sure you wash your hands afterward before touching anything, especially your eyes). Season with salt and pepper.

3. Bake for about 20 minutes, checking on them to prevent burning and flipping halfway through the cooking time.

4. Remove from the oven, sprinkle the lime juice over them, and serve with Chimichurri (if using).

VARIATION 1 **MAPLE-CINNAMON SWEET POTATO FRIES:** Make a sweeter version by drizzling the sweet potato wedges with 2 tablespoons maple syrup and ¼ to ½ teaspoon ground cinnamon. Follow the rest of the recipe as written.

VARIATION 2 **PLAIN SWEET POTATO FRIES:** Skip the cayenne and lime juice, and just season with salt and pepper.

PALEO PAIR: Serve as a side with Burger Bowls (page 51).

SWEET POTATO CHIPS

I buy sweet potato chips all the time from Trader Joe's, but I know they're cooked in non-Paleo oils and usually loaded with preservatives, so whenever I can, I make them myself. This recipe is a good one, although it does have a long cook time. Here, they're cooked low and slow as opposed to high and fast because to get them crunchy, they need to be thin, but to keep them from burning, they need to cook slowly. It's worth it. (You could do them for 25 minutes at 400°F; if you do, just be mindful and check on them frequently.) **SERVES 2 TO 4**

PREP TIME: 15 minutes
COOK TIME: 2 hours

NF **V**

2 large sweet potatoes, thinly sliced with a knife or mandolin

2 tablespoons extra-virgin olive oil

Salt

Freshly ground black pepper

1. Preheat the oven to 250°F.

2. In a large bowl, toss the sweet potato slices with the olive oil. Pour them out onto one or two large baking sheets in a single layer, and season with salt and pepper.

3. Bake for 1½ to 2 hours, checking on them after 30 minutes. At the halfway point, check them again to prevent burning, and flip them.

4. Serve warm or at room temperature.

VARIATION 1 **GARLIC SWEET POTATO CHIPS:** Season the chips with 1 or 2 teaspoons garlic powder before baking.

VARIATION 2 **CINNAMON-HONEY SWEET POTATO CHIPS:** Season with ½ teaspoon ground cinnamon, and drizzle with 1 or 2 tablespoons honey before baking.

PALEO PAIR: Dip these in Ranch Dressing (page 75) or Not-Spinach Artichoke Dip (page 117).

CURRIED SWEET POTATOES

Mashed sweet potatoes are delicious, but they can get boring pretty quickly. Enter curried sweet potatoes, a slightly mashed recipe that's full of exciting flavors like curry and cinnamon. This recipe is great for days when you don't feel like experimenting much in the kitchen but want something just a bit different. **SERVES 4**

PREP TIME: 10 minutes
COOK TIME: 15 minutes

4 medium sweet potatoes, peeled and cubed

2 tablespoons ghee

½ onion, diced

2 garlic cloves, minced

1½ teaspoons curry powder

½ teaspoon ground cinnamon

⅛ teaspoon red pepper flakes or ground cayenne pepper

Salt

Freshly ground black pepper

⅓ cup canned full-fat coconut milk

1. In a large saucepan filled with boiling water over medium-high heat, cook the sweet potatoes until fork-tender, about 15 minutes.

2. With about 5 minutes to go on the potatoes, melt the ghee in another large saucepan. Sauté the onion and garlic until the sweet potatoes are done.

3. Drain the potatoes, and mash them with a fork. Add them to the pan with the onion and garlic, and stir. Season with the curry powder, cinnamon, red pepper flakes, salt, and pepper. Add the coconut milk and stir. Serve warm.

VARIATION 1 **CUBED CURRIED SWEET POTATOES:** To speed up this recipe, instead of mashing the sweet potatoes, add them to the pot diced or cubed. Serve in a bowl with the sauce poured over them. Garnish with a handful of sliced scallions or chopped fresh parsley.

VARIATION 2 **CURRY ROASTED SWEET POTATOES:** Toss cubed sweet potatoes in a bowl with 2 tablespoons olive oil and the spices listed in the original recipe. Roast at 400°F for 20 to 25 minutes, or until fork-tender.

PALEO PAIR: Serve beneath a bowl of Shrimp Stir-Fry (page 96).

BAKED SWEET POTATOES

Baking a sweet potato is one of the easiest ways you can prepare the tough root vegetable—it may take an hour, but all you do is pop it in the oven and set a timer. I love making them as a side for dinner, so long as I remember that I had planned to make them so I don't end up having to postpone dinnertime by an hour. Make yourself a note, and throw them in the oven as soon as you get home from work. **SERVES 4**

PREP TIME: 5 minutes
COOK TIME: 1 hour

NF V

4 sweet potatoes

1. Preheat the oven to 400°F.

2. Poke each sweet potato 6 or 7 times with a fork. Place them on a baking sheet and bake until tender, 45 minutes to 1 hour, and serve.

VARIATION 1 **BAKED SWEET POTATOES WITH GARLIC BUTTER AND CHIVES:** In a small bowl, mix 3 or 4 tablespoons room-temperature butter with 1 or 2 cloves finely minced garlic. Mix well, and add a dollop to each baked sweet potato. Garnish with chopped fresh chives, and season with salt and pepper.

VARIATION 2 **MAPLE-COCONUT SWEET POTATOES:** Top each baked sweet potato with a drizzle of maple syrup and a pinch of unsweetened shredded coconut. Add 1/8 teaspoon ground cinnamon to each, if desired.

PALEO PAIR: Serve baked sweet potatoes with Chicken, Steak, and Shrimp Kebabs (page 98).

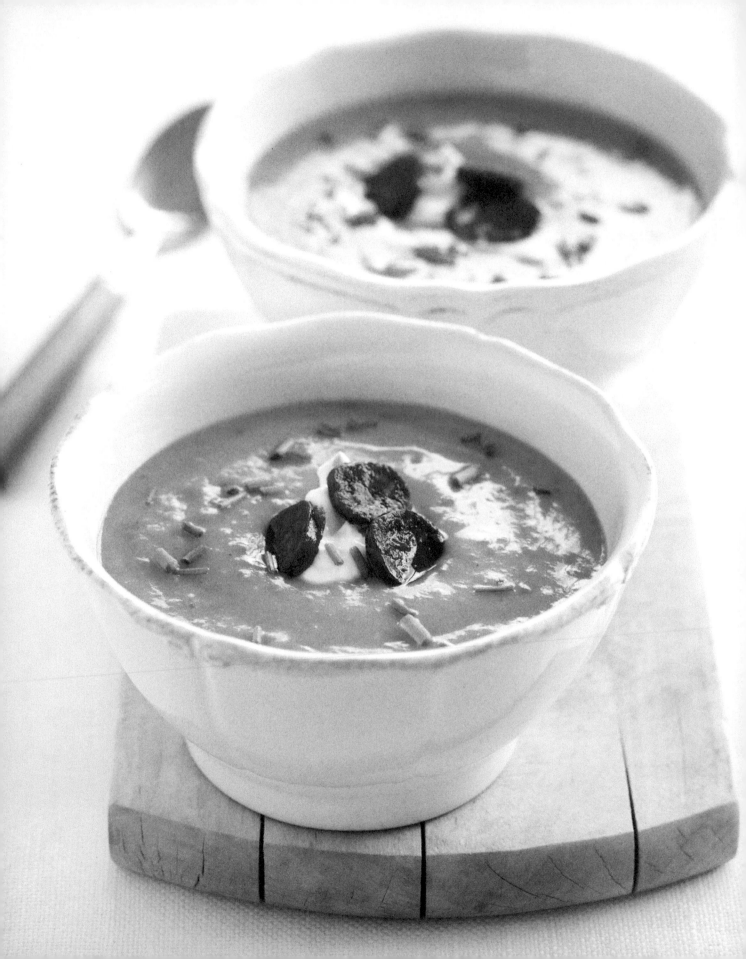

SWEET POTATO SOUP WITH CHORIZO AND COCONUT CREAM

This soup is rich and flavorful, made with roasted sweet potatoes and chorizo and then mixed with full-fat coconut milk for the rich creaminess that you look for in a thick soup or bisque. It's perfect on a chilly fall or winter day for lunch with a simple kale salad, or you can serve it as a first course at your next dinner party. For added convenience, make ahead and reheat. **SERVES 4 TO 6**

PREP TIME: 10 minutes
COOK TIME: 60 minutes

NF

4 sweet potatoes, peeled and cubed

2 tablespoons extra-virgin olive oil

2 tablespoons grass-fed butter

3 garlic cloves, chopped

1 onion, chopped

2 dried bay leaves

5 cups chicken broth

1 pound chorizo, sliced

1 (13.5-ounce) can full-fat coconut milk, refrigerated (reserve 2 to 3 tablespoons for garnish)

2 tablespoons chopped fresh chives, for garnish

PREP TIP: Always keep a can of coconut milk in your fridge. Whenever I start cooking a recipe that calls for coconut cream, I'm always in trouble; because it's a canned product, I keep forgetting that it needs to be refrigerated overnight to get the cream off the top. If you just keep a can in the fridge at all times, you'll always be ready for any recipe that calls for it!

1. Preheat the oven to 400°F.

2. On a large roasting pan, drizzle the sweet potatoes with the olive oil, and roast until browned and fork-tender, 25 to 30 minutes.

3. While the sweet potatoes are cooking, in a large saucepan over low heat, melt the butter. Sauté the garlic and onions for 10 minutes. Add the roasted sweet potatoes, bay leaves, and broth, and raise the heat to medium-high. Bring to a low boil, reduce the heat to low, and simmer for 10 minutes.

4. In a small skillet, cook the chorizo until crispy, 5 to 7 minutes.

5. Remove the soup from the heat, and add about ⅓ cup of the cream from the top of the refrigerated can of coconut milk (leave a few tablespoons for topping). Stir well, and carefully purée the soup using either an immersion blender or countertop blender. (If using a countertop blender, blend in batches and hold a clean dishtowel over the lid while blending to avoid hot soup eruptions.)

6. In a small bowl, beat the extra coconut cream with a whisk or hand mixer until fluffy.

7. Pour the soup into serving bowls, and top with whipped coconut cream and 3 to 4 pieces each of crispy chorizo. Garnish with the chives, and serve.

VARIATION 1 **SPICY SWEET POTATO SOUP:** Add ¼ to ½ teaspoon red pepper flakes to the soup, depending on how spicy you'd like it to be.

VARIATION 2 **SWEET POTATO SOUP WITH BACON:** If you can't find (or don't like) chorizo, fry 3 or 4 slices bacon and chop them up for the soup topping.

BBQ-STUFFED SWEET POTATOES

These sweet potatoes topped with pulled pork are sweet and tangy, and they make a great, easy weeknight dinner, as long as you've prepped a few things ahead of time (the pork, for example). All you then have to do is throw together a quick salad, and you have a pretty complete meal that's ready to go. **SERVES 4**

PREP TIME: 10 minutes
COOK TIME: 1 hour, 30 minutes

4 sweet potatoes

1 pound Pulled Pork BBQ (page 74)

BBQ Sauce (page 131), for drizzling or dipping

1 to 2 tablespoons thinly sliced red onion or scallions, for garnish

1. Preheat the oven to 400°F.

2. Poke each sweet potato 6 or 7 times with a fork. Place them on a baking sheet, and bake until tender, 45 minutes to 1 hour.

3. Remove them from the oven, and slice a big wedge out of the top of each. Reserve the wedges for dipping into extra BBQ Sauce.

4. Divide the Pulled Pork BBQ among the sweet potatoes by filling the gap left by the wedges you cut, and drizzle with BBQ Sauce.

5. Serve garnished with red onion or scallions, with extra BBQ Sauce on the side.

VARIATION 1 **CARNITAS-STUFFED SWEET POTATOES:** Stuff baked sweet potatoes with Carnitas (page 69) instead of Pulled Pork BBQ for a different version of this recipe. Bake as directed.

VARIATION 2 **VEGETARIAN STUFFED SWEET POTATOES:** Top baked sweet potatoes with a big scoop of Perfect Sautéed Mushrooms (page 207) instead of meat.

PREP TIP: Make the pulled pork in the slow cooker the night before the day you want to make this recipe, so all you have to do is bake the sweet potatoes.

ROASTED SWEET POTATOES

This is the classic way to prepare sweet potatoes, in my opinion. It's so simple, and you can serve it with almost any protein plus a green vegetable, and you have a complete Paleo dinner without having to do much planning. It's like the Emergency Pasta (page 154) of Paleo carbs, if you will. **SERVES 4**

PREP TIME: 5 minutes
COOK TIME: 35 minutes

NF **V**

4 sweet potatoes, peeled and chopped

1 onion, quartered and divided

2 garlic cloves, minced

3 or 4 tablespoons extra-virgin olive oil

1. Preheat the oven to 425°F.

2. In a large bowl, toss the sweet potatoes with the onion, garlic, and olive oil.

3. Transfer to a baking sheet, and roast for 30 to 35 minutes, or until the sweet potatoes are fork-tender and slightly browned, and serve.

VARIATION 1 **BALSAMIC-ROASTED SWEET POTATOES:** Toss the sweet potatoes, onion, garlic, and olive oil with ¼ cup Balsamic Vinaigrette (page 89). Continue with the recipe as written.

VARIATION 2 **SPICY ROASTED SWEET POTATOES:** After transferring the sweet potatoes to a baking sheet, sprinkle with ¼ teaspoon ground cayenne pepper. Continue with the recipe as written.

PALEO PAIR: Serve as a side with Carnitas (page 69) for dinner.

TWICE-BAKED SWEET POTATOES

These twice-baked sweet potatoes are super easy to customize so you can make them again and again and not feel like you're always serving or eating the same thing. Sweet potatoes are always good, but if you're constantly just roasting them and serving them with chicken (I'm really guilty of that one), after a while you start feeling like Paleo is boring. If you've made it to this point in this book, I hope you know that is *not* true! **SERVES 4**

PREP TIME: 15 minutes
COOK TIME: 1 hour, 20 minutes

NF

4 medium sweet potatoes

6 tablespoons grass-fed butter, at room temperature

1 garlic clove, minced

5 or 6 scallions, sliced, divided

1 (13.5-ounce) can full-fat coconut milk, refrigerated

4 slices bacon, cooked and chopped, divided

Salt

Freshly ground black pepper

1. Preheat the oven to 400°F.

2. Poke each sweet potato 6 or 7 times with a fork. Place them on a baking sheet, and bake until tender, 45 minutes to 1 hour. Remove them from the oven, and reduce the oven temperature to 375°F.

3. Cut the sweet potatoes in half, and scoop out most of the insides with a spoon (you want to leave a thin layer of flesh so the skins don't rip). Transfer the sweet potato flesh to a medium bowl, and line up the skins on the baking sheet.

4. In the bowl with the flesh, mix it with the butter, garlic, half the scallions, and the coconut cream from the top of the can of coconut milk. Fold in three-quarters of the chopped bacon, and season with salt and pepper. Spoon the filling into the sweet potato skins.

5. Bake for 15 to 20 minutes, or until warmed through.

6. Garnish with the remaining bacon and the rest of the scallions, and serve.

VARIATION 1 **TWICE-BAKED SWEET POTATOES WITH SAUSAGE:** Instead of bacon, add ¼ pound cooked spicy Italian sausage to the sweet potato filling.

VARIATION 2 **DESSERT TWICE-BAKED SWEET POTATOES:** Instead of garlic and scallions, mix ½ cup shredded coconut, ¼ cup raisins, 2 tablespoons maple syrup, and 1 teaspoon ground cinnamon with the coconut milk for the filling.

PREP TIP: Make this recipe through step 4 (fill the sweet potato skins), and then cover and refrigerate until ready to bake. Bake about half an hour before ready to serve.

SWEET POTATO CASSEROLE WITH WALNUTS AND CRISPY ONIONS

This sweet potato casserole is a flavorful side dish. The crispy, savory onions are almost like Paleo onion rings, and they pair really well with the extra unexpected crunch of the walnuts and the sweetness of the potatoes. **SERVES 4 TO 6**

PREP TIME: 15 minutes
COOK TIME: 35 minutes

6 sweet potatoes, peeled and chopped

1 large onion

1 egg, whisked

½ cup tapioca flour

½ cup almond flour

2 tablespoons grass-fed butter

3 garlic cloves, minced

1 (13.5-ounce) can full-fat coconut milk

Salt

Freshly ground black pepper

1 cup walnuts

PREP TIP: Make this casserole ahead of time, and bake before serving in a 350°F oven for 20 to 30 minutes.

1. Preheat the oven to 400°F.

2. In a large saucepan, boil the sweet potatoes in enough water to cover them for 15 minutes, or until fork-tender. Drain well, and set aside.

3. While the potatoes are boiling, spiralize or slice the onion, and dip it into a small bowl containing the whisked egg. Put the tapioca flour in one dish and the almond flour in another, and batter the onion by removing it piece by piece from the egg bowl, dipping each piece first into the tapioca flour and then into the almond flour. (If you're short on time, you can put the onion and both flours in a large zip-top bag and shake it.) Set aside.

4. In a large sauté pan over medium heat, melt the butter. Sauté the garlic for 2 to 3 minutes before adding the sweet potatoes. Mash the potatoes (they don't have to be perfectly smooth) with a spoon or handheld mixer, and add the coconut milk. Season with salt and pepper.

5. Transfer the potatoes to an 8-by-12-inch baking dish, and top with the walnuts and onions. Bake for 10 to 15 minutes, just until warmed through and the onions are crispy, and serve.

VARIATION 1 **SAUSAGE-SWEET POTATO CASSEROLE:** Cook 1 pound spicy Italian sausage in a sauté pan until browned, about 10 minutes. Add to the bottom of the baking dish as a first layer. Continue with the recipe as written.

VARIATION 2 **DESSERT SWEET POTATO CASSEROLE:** Skip the onions, garlic, salt, and pepper, and season the mashed sweet potato with ½ tablespoon ground cinnamon and ¼ cup maple syrup or honey when you add the coconut milk. Top with the walnuts as in the original recipe, and garnish with a handful unsweetened coconut flakes.

SWEET POTATO HASH BROWNS

I make these sweet potato hash browns every time we have weekend guests, and it's always a hit. Sometimes it can be hard to get sweet potatoes as crispy as you want them to be, but for some reason, this recipe always delivers on flavor and texture. Ghee works to our advantage because of its high smoke point, so don't be afraid to cook them on medium-high to high heat. They're delicious with eggs or even just on their own with a side of bacon or sausage. Any leftovers are great reheated for lunch, too. **SERVES 4 TO 6**

PREP TIME: 10 minutes
COOK TIME: 25 minutes

NF

2 tablespoons ghee

¼ cup chopped onions

1 garlic clove, chopped

2 or 3 sweet potatoes, diced

Salt

Freshly ground black pepper

¼ cup chopped green bell pepper

1. In a large sauté pan over medium heat, melt the ghee. Cook the onion and garlic until the onion is slightly translucent, about 5 minutes.

2. Add the sweet potatoes to the pan, and give it a good stir to cover all the pieces with ghee. Season with salt and pepper.

3. Raise the heat to medium-high, and cook for 15 to 20 minutes, or until the sweet potatoes begin to brown on all sides and get crispy. With about 5 minutes of cooking time left, add the bell pepper.

4. Serve immediately.

VARIATION 1 **SHREDDED SWEET POTATO HASH BROWNS:** For a different texture, you can shred the sweet potatoes. Continue with the recipe as written, but the cook time may be a minute or two less since the shredded sweet potatoes will be thinner.

VARIATION 2 **SWEET POTATO–SQUASH HASH BROWNS:** Add 1 cup peeled and diced butternut squash to the recipe if it's in season and you want to make this an even heartier dish.

PALEO PAIR: Serve as a side with Baked Eggs in Tomato Sauce (page 22) for a complete breakfast or brunch.

PANTRY BASIC: DRY RUB

This is the dry rub we use whenever we make Baby Back Ribs (page 70)—it's so good. You can mix it all up ahead of time and then add fresh orange zest as needed. It's also great as a seasoning for chicken, shrimp, beef, or pretty much any protein. **MAKES ¼ CUP**

PREP TIME: 5 minutes
COOK TIME: None

30 **NF** **V**

2 teaspoons ground paprika

1½ teaspoons salt

1 teaspoon chili powder

1 teaspoon onion powder

1 teaspoon freshly ground black pepper

¾ teaspoon freshly ground white pepper

½ teaspoon ground cayenne pepper

½ teaspoon ground coriander

½ teaspoon ground cumin

½ teaspoon garlic powder

¼ teaspoon ground cinnamon

Zest of 1 orange

1. In a mason jar or other container with a tightly fitting lid, shake or mix to combine the paprika, salt, chili powder, onion powder, black and white pepper, cayenne pepper, coriander, cumin, garlic powder, and cinnamon.

2. Add the freshly grated orange zest when you want to use the rub.

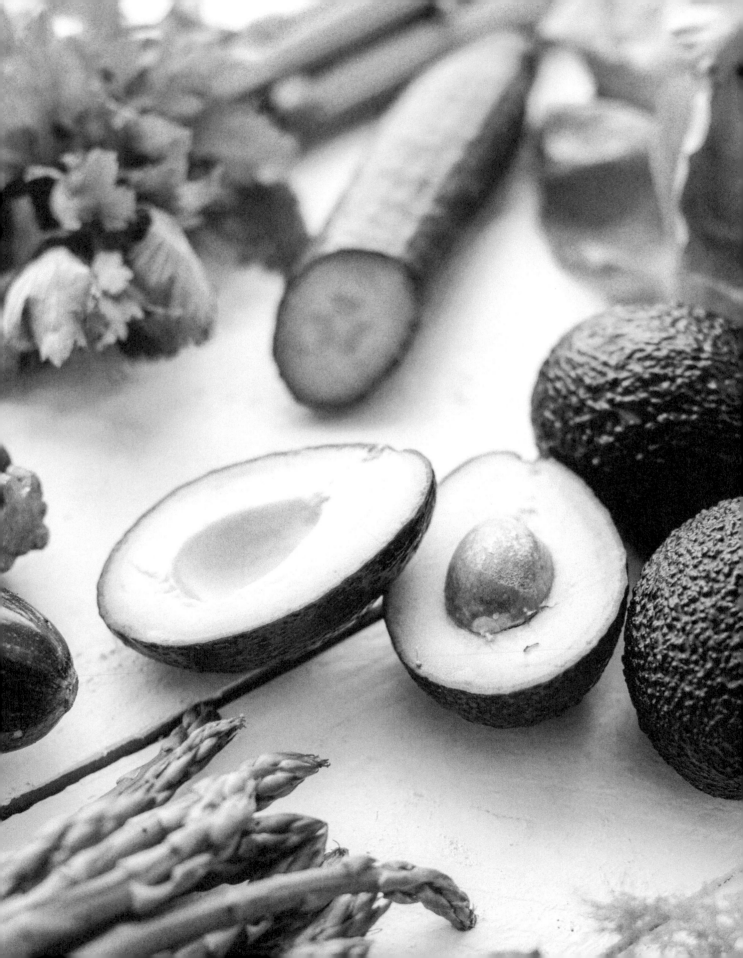

The Dirty Dozen and
the Clean Fifteen

A nonprofit environmental watchdog organization called Environmental Working Group (EWG) looks at data supplied by the U.S. Department of Agriculture (USDA) and the Food and Drug Administration (FDA) about pesticide residues. Each year it compiles a list of the best and worst pesticide loads found in commercial crops. You can use these lists to decide which fruits and vegetables to buy organic to minimize your exposure to pesticides and which produce is considered safe enough to buy conventionally. This does not mean they are pesticide-free, though, so wash these fruits and vegetables thoroughly.

2016 DIRTY DOZEN

Apples	Nectarines
Celery	Peaches
Cherries	Spinach
Cherry tomatoes	Strawberries
Cucumbers	Sweet bell peppers
Grapes	Tomatoes

In addition to the Dirty Dozen, the EWG added two types of produce contaminated with highly toxic organo-phosphate insecticides:

Kale/collard greens	Hot peppers

2016 CLEAN FIFTEEN

Asparagus	Pineapples
Avocados	Sweet corn
Cabbage	Sweet peas (frozen)
Cantaloupes	
Cauliflower	
Eggplant	
Grapefruit	
Honeydew Melon	
Kiwi	
Mango	
Onions	
Papayas	

Measurements and Conversion Tables

VOLUME EQUIVALENTS (LIQUID)

STANDARD	US STANDARD (OUNCES)	METRIC (APPROXIMATE)
2 tablespoons	1 fl. oz.	30 mL
¼ cup	2 fl. oz.	60 mL
½ cup	4 fl. oz.	120 mL
1 cup	8 fl. oz.	240 mL
1½ cups	12 fl. oz.	355 mL
2 cups or 1 pint	16 fl. oz.	475 mL
4 cups or 1 quart	32 fl. oz.	1 L
1 gallon	128 fl. oz.	4 L

OVEN TEMPERATURES

FAHRENHEIT (F)	CELSIUS (C) (APPROXIMATE)
250°	120°
300°	150°
325°	165°
350°	180°
375°	190°
400°	200°
425°	220°
450°	230°

VOLUME EQUIVALENTS (DRY)

STANDARD	METRIC (APPROXIMATE)
⅛ teaspoon	0.5 mL
¼ teaspoon	1 mL
½ teaspoon	2 mL
¾ teaspoon	4 mL
1 teaspoon	5 mL
1 tablespoon	15 mL
¼ cup	59 mL
⅓ cup	79 mL
½ cup	118 mL
⅔ cup	156 mL
¾ cup	177 mL
1 cup	235 mL
2 cups or 1 pint	475 mL
3 cups	700 mL
4 cups or 1 quart	1 L

WEIGHT EQUIVALENTS

STANDARD	METRIC (APPROXIMATE)
½ ounce	15 g
1 ounce	30 g
2 ounces	60 g
4 ounces	115 g
8 ounces	225 g
12 ounces	340 g
16 ounces or 1 pound	455 g

Resources

- **Robb Wolf**
  robbwolf.com
  Widely regarded as an expert in all things Paleo, Robb Wolf is a great person to start with. His blog has lots of practical issues and solutions, and he does a great job going over the science of Paleo and why it can be an exceptionally beneficial diet.

- **Whole 30**
  whole30.com
  I've never done a Whole 30 but do think it can be a great place to start if you're feeling unsure or overwhelmed about changing your diet. The community is great and has lots of meal ideas and inspiration on the site, as well as their Instagram feeds (@whole30 and @whole30recipes).

- **Paleo Subreddit**
  reddit.com/r/paleo
  A great forum for sharing stories and asking questions. I was on here all the time when I first started out. Take everything with a grain of salt—most advice you will encounter is through experience and not necessarily expertise, but I have always found it really helpful.

Acknowledgements

This book happened quickly and wouldn't have been possible without the help of quite a few people.

First is my mom, for introducing me to Paleo when she did, for being the kind of cook who encourages creativity and experimentation, for Paleo-ifying so many of my favorite recipes, and for being so incredibly generous in everything that she does for me.

Thank you, Sean, for being the kind of brother and friend whom I could call on at any time of day for recipe inspiration. You are a better cook than I will ever be and I'm so proud to be your sister.

Thanks to my dad for always being a reassuring source of support, and for encouraging my writing and creativity from the beginning.

I can't thank Callisto Media enough. Writing a book has been a dream of mine since I learned to read, and you handed me that opportunity—and it has truly touched me. Thank you so much.

Thank you to my blog readers and the readers of this book for making my life and career such a joy. It is truly an honor to be able to reach out and interact with so many people all over the world. I hope this book of recipes is exactly what you're looking for.

Thank you Dwight Schrute for your enthusiasm when it comes to beets. That chapter is for you, no matter how fictional you may be.

Last but certainly not least, thanks go to my amazing husband Rob, who is patient when I'm overwhelmed, encouraging when I'm tired, and kind and sweet and silly every day. Thank you for always investing in my dreams, and for being one of them yourself.

About the Author

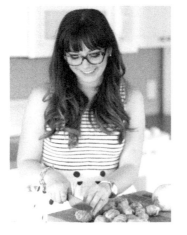

Megan Flynn Peterson is the writer behind Freckled Italian, a blog that focuses on life, love, personal style, nostalgia, and lots of food. With a master's degree in children's literature and an affinity for cultural studies, good food, wine, bookstores, and changing seasons, Megan doesn't sit still for long. She has lived in California, Virginia, Minnesota, and North Carolina; and currently considers home to be wherever her husband and their rescue dog are. She discovered Paleo in 2012 and hasn't looked back. This is her first cookbook.

You can read more from Megan at freckleditalian.com, or find her on Instagram and Twitter @mflynnpete.

Index